Come from Away

NURSES WHO IMMIGRATED TO NEWFOUNDLAND AND LABRADOR

JEANETTE WALSH ✳ MARILYN BEATON

Library and Archives Canada Cataloguing in Publication

Walsh, Jeanette, 1944-
Come from away : nurses who immigrated to Newfoundland and Labrador /
Jeanette Walsh & Marilyn Beaton.
ISBN 978-1-55081-359-3
1. Nursing--Newfoundland and Labrador--History. 2. Nurses--Newfoundland and
Labrador--Interviews. 3. Nurses--Newfoundland and Labrador--Biography.
4. Oral history--Newfoundland and Labrador. I. Beaton, Marilyn, 1947- II. Title.
RT6.N48W34 2011   610.7309718   C2011-905065-X

Canada Council   Conseil des Arts   Canada   Newfoundland
for the Arts   du Canada   Labrador

Breakwater Books acknowledges the support of the Canada Council for the Arts which
last year invested $20.1 million in writing and publishing throughout Canada.
We acknowledge the Government of Canada through the Canada Book Fund and the
Government of Newfoundland and Labrador through the Department of Tourism,
Culture and Recreation for our publishing activities.
PRINTED AND BOUND IN CANADA.

Dedication

THIS BOOK IS DEDICATED TO THE MANY NURSES
WHO IMMIGRATED TO THE PROVINCE, PARTICULARLY THOSE
WHO STAYED, FOR THEIR CONTRIBUTION TO NURSING
AND HEALTH CARE AND THEIR COMMITMENT TO THE PEOPLE
OF NEWFOUNDLAND AND LABRADOR.

Contents

List of Acronyms

ARNNL:	Association of Registered Nurses of Newfoundland and Labrador
BN:	Bachelor of Nursing
CNA:	Colonial Nurse Association
GP:	General Practitioner
HR:	Human Resources
ICU:	Intensive Care Unit
IGA:	International Grenfell Association
IV:	Intravenous (injection)
MUN:	Memorial University of Newfoundland
NONIA:	Newfoundland Outport Nursing and Industrial Association
OBS:	Obstetrics
ONA:	Overseas Nursing Association
ONC:	Outport Nursing Committee
OR:	Operating Room
RGN:	Registered Graduate Nurse
RN:	Registered Nurse
RT:	Radio Telephone; can refer to equipment, personnel, or the division
SCM:	State Certified Midwife
SRN:	State Registered Nurse

❋

Introduction

OVERSEAS RECRUITMENT OF NURSES has been part of nursing and health care in Newfoundland and Labrador since Wilfred Grenfell brought the first two nurses to Labrador in 1893. Although there is no known record of an exact number, hundreds of nurses came to the province to work since that time. (Newfoundland was a country until 1949, when it joined Canada and became a province. Its name was officially changed to Newfoundland and Labrador in 2001, but in this book we refer to it as such for its full provincial history.) The majority worked the period of their contract and returned home, but many stayed.

The contribution of these overseas nurses to nursing and health care in Newfoundland and Labrador is a significant, but undocumented, piece of the province's history. As told through their compelling accounts, these nurses encountered challenges in the workplace and most found themselves living in a place with a very foreign lifestyle, culture, and climate. However, those who stayed adapted and even thrived, and in many cases spent their entire career serving the people of Newfoundland and Labrador.

This nursing history project was intended to document the recollections of nurses who immigrated to Newfoundland and Labrador and opted to stay. The interviews conducted for this project focused on why the individuals chose to come, what they knew about the province, what they had to do to get here, what challenges they encountered in their practice and with the lifestyle and culture, and why they stayed. In addition to sharing their experiences, the nurses also revealed much about the living and socio-economic conditions in the province in the early 1950s and beyond, particularly in northern Newfoundland and coastal Labrador. They were very candid in telling both personal and professional stories. In choosing what to include from the interviews in this book, we decided to stay with the original purpose of the project outlined in the previous questions.

Not surprisingly, there were common experiences among the group— requirements for immigration and nursing licences, for example—and these are discussed in general terms with variations included in individual stories. We acknowledge that the nurses' recollections around their immigration experience may not always be historically accurate, but accept that the stories reflect their genuine memories.

The nurses were recruited through our personal contacts or were identified by other participants. Forty-one nurses who immigrated to Newfoundland and Labrador between 1949 and 2007 were interviewed. They came to work as community nurses in rural areas, as staff nurses in community and urban hospitals, and in nursing stations along the coast of Labrador. Twenty-seven nurses came from the United Kingdom, with the remaining from Ireland, Switzerland, Sierra Leone, Nigeria, Philippines, United States, Denmark, Kenya, and Vietnam. Thirty were State Registered Nurses (SRN) and thirty-two completed midwifery as State Certified Midwives (SCM), training considered an asset for nurses planning to travel. Nineteen were recruited by the International Grenfell Association (IGA) to work in northern Newfoundland and coastal Labrador.

The most common reason for immigrating was the opportunity for travel and adventure, although several were motivated by the work of Wilfred Grenfell, who set up the Grenfell Mission in 1892 to counter the complete lack of health care services he had discovered in New-foundland and Labrador. Many nurses learned of job opportunities through advertisements in British nursing magazines. Immigration to Canada required that nurses have a passport, a work permit or visa, Registered Nurse (RN) equivalency, a medical examination, references, a police screening, an employment interview, and a job. Applicants were screened by Canadian Immigration. The time to process a nurse's application varied from several months to several years and was often influenced by the need for nurses. Eligibility to immigrate was based on a points system, with points awarded for specific factors such as occupation. Newfoundland and Labrador employers could recruit overseas only if there were no Canadian nurses available to fill local positions. Overseas nurses received work visas if they had a specific skill not common to North American nursing graduates, such as midwifery, or if there was a shortage of nurses in Canada.

Nurses recruited to Newfoundland and Labrador were expected to commit to a specific work period, which varied depending on the employer's needs. In the 1950s, the duration was two to three years, whereas in times of nursing shortages, the duration might be as little as three to four months. Outside of a specified work period, other conditions of employment were not always clear, which occasionally resulted in different work expectations for overseas nurses as compared to local nurses. In one situation, recruited nurses were hired for a 10-month contract only to discover, upon their arrival, that they were required to work six days per week while local nurses worked five days per week. In some cases, nurses arrived to find they had been assigned, without consultation, to a different location or nursing unit than what they had signed on for. It was a case of "go where we need you."

All nurses had to be eligible for a licence to practice nursing and were required to meet Registered Nurse (RN) equivalency, which meant they had to have comparable education and practice experiences as nurses educated in the province. Overseas nurses submitted their professional qualifications to the Association of Registered Nurses of Newfoundland and Labrador (ARNNL) for evaluation. If they met the minimal requirements to practice nursing in the province, they were issued a licence. However, provincial nursing programs included obstetrics (OBS) and psychiatry, whereas some overseas nurses had only OBS or only psychiatry. In those cases they were required to complete a program of studies and write the RN exam in the deficient area. When Newfoundland and Labrador adopted the Canadian RN exam in the late 1970s, overseas nurses were required to write it. In both cases, nurses were issued a temporary licence until they passed the RN exam, which had to be written within a specified time frame. While working on a temporary licence they were paid as graduate nurses. When they passed the RN exam, they were registered with ARNNL and paid accordingly.

Nurses were offered few incentives; their airfare was paid to Newfoundland and Labrador, and if they worked the term of the contract, their return airfare was paid. In most cases accommodations were subsidized. In some cases, uniforms were provided, but not always, and given the different professional dress codes between their home country and North America, many had to purchase uniforms. Up to the late 1980s, some were attracted by higher salaries than those in the UK, along with a much lower cost of living.

The majority had no idea about the place to which they were coming. Many emigrated from England, with a population of approximately 51 million across 50,000 square miles, to a province with a population of slightly more than one-half million across 110,000 square miles. No wonder so many were overwhelmed by the vastness of Newfoundland and Labrador!

A great number came from large teaching hospitals in London that had up to 1,200 beds. The largest hospital in Newfoundland and Labrador had approximately 500 beds, so understandably the nurses encountered differences in nursing practice. They felt the practice setting was more informal than at home, as was the relationship between the various levels of nurses and physicians. They felt Newfoundland and Labrador nurses worked harder but had less autonomy and independence in their practice. Particular frustrations included having to get a doctor's order for activities accepted as a nursing responsibility in the UK, and the method of medication administration.

Most of the nurses came to Newfoundland and Labrador because it was part of an English-speaking country, only to have great difficulty comprehending the local dialects and different terminology for everyday things, which could be confounding but also resulted in some funny encounters.

In rural areas, local nurses were welcoming and helpful. The new nurse was a novelty in the community, as often the nurse was the only health care provider and subsequently was held in high esteem. The people were generally very accepting and drew the nurse into community life. In urban areas, overseas nurses were often left to fend for themselves. Many had difficulty coming from an anonymous society to one in which everybody knew everybody else, and knew what was happening in the community.

The most common reason overseas nurses stayed was marriage, and those who married automatically received landed immigrant status. Most had developed strong feelings about the province and identified many positives about living here. Some returned home at the end of their contract but found the practice environment in Britain less satisfying and more highly pressured than in Newfoundland and Labrador. Most indicated they enjoyed a better standard of living and better lifestyle than what they had at home. Those with children saw them as providing roots in the province and felt it was a safer environment in which to rear children. Most maintained a strong connection to "home," with visits to their family every other year along with regular family visits to Newfoundland and Labrador.

This book shares the stories of 41 nurses who immigrated to Newfoundland and Labrador and opted to make a life and career here. Their stories span five decades and shed light on the challenges they encountered adapting to nursing and life in Newfoundland and Labrador, along with the tremendous contribution they made to nursing and health care in the province. The stories are funny, poignant, and highlight the courage and commitment of these nurses, reaffirming the important contribution nurses have made to health care in Newfoundland and Labrador.

Section One

IMMIGRATION TO URBAN AND RURAL AREAS
OF THE ISLAND OF NEWFOUNDLAND

Introduction

RECRUITMENT TO URBAN AND RURAL AREAS

THE COLONIAL NURSE ASSOCIATION (CNA) was a private nurse recruitment agency that sent nursing sisters across the British Empire and recruited nurses based on the personal judgments of the selection committee about the nurse's class, age, training, personal attributes, manners and characteristics. In existence from 1896, it was renamed the Overseas Nursing Association (ONA) in 1919. In the 1920s and 1930s, overseas recruitment focused on nurses for outport communities in Newfoundland and Labrador. Nurses graduating from programs in St. John's were either employed by their training hospital or in private duty. Also, their program did not prepare them to work in rural areas, so very few opted to work there. In 1920 Lady Harris, wife of the British appointed governor, used ONA to recruit six nurse midwives for isolated Newfoundland communities where there were no medical services. The government agreed to pay half the nurses' salaries if the committee provided the rest through fund-raising efforts. Patients paid one dollar annually. Six nurses were hired from England on two-year contracts and were posted in regions across the island. At the end of their contract in 1922, four returned to England. The new governor's wife decided to restructure the Outport Nursing Committee (ONC) so that outport women would be hired to knit and weave goods to be sold to the public with the profits used to support the nurses' salaries. In 1924, the ONC became NONIA: the Newfoundland Outport

Nursing and Industrial Association. (Higgins, J. 2008. Health Care Organizations under the Commission of Government, Newfoundland and Labrador, pp. 1–6. http://www.heritage.nf.ca/society/cghealth_org.html).

ONA was also used by NONIA to recruit nurses until the mid-1930s. It recruited nurses for outport Newfoundland until 1934, when the Newfoundland government assumed responsibility for all rural nursing services in the country. The eight nurses working with NONIA at that time were transferred to the Newfoundland Department of Health and Public Welfare, while the industrial section continues under the NONIA trademark to this day.

District nurses, known today as Community Health Nurses, were the sole health care providers to large groups of isolated communities in rural Newfoundland and had only radio or telegraph contact with a doctor. Many of these nurses were recruited from overseas. In 1935, the Newfoundland government opened a series of cottage hospitals across the island and overseas nurses were also recruited to staff them. District nurses continued to be the predominant health care providers but now, because of the cottage hospitals, they had greater access to a physician or a health care facility. The government continued to use ONA to recruit nurses for cottage hospitals and as district nurses in Newfoundland outports until ONA ended in 1966.

In St. John's in the early 1950s, hospitals began to experience nursing shortages as a result of changes in the nursing education programs. Up to this point student nurses comprised the majority of nursing staff in city hospitals. When classroom content was increased, additional registered nurses were needed to staff the hospitals and again overseas recruitment became the primary method to obtain these nurses. When the new school of nursing began at Memorial University of Newfoundland in St. John's in the mid-1960s, overseas recruitment was used to obtain qualified teaching faculty for the Baccalaureate in

Nursing program. In rural Newfoundland and Labrador, nursing shortages continued to create a need for overseas recruitment until the mid-1980s. Since the 1990s, the focus of overseas recruitment has been recruitment of midwives for northern Newfoundland and Labrador, where they are permitted to practice.

Early nurses coming to Newfoundland and Labrador were white, English speaking women from a more sophisticated, richer society with a more advanced health care system than that which existed in the province. Most graduated from large teaching hospitals in the UK that were more advanced than those in Newfoundland and Labrador, particularly in the early years of nurse recruitment. Given its Commonwealth ties to the UK, it is not surprising that the province looked to Britain to recruit nurses.

Jean Lewis, a nurse manager involved with overseas recruitment for the island of Newfoundland, tells us how the government and hospitals were able to find and attract nurses to this side of the Atlantic. She went to Britain "to interview nurses for Waterford Hospital [the psychiatric hospital] and the General Hospital" and recalls:

"But my main focus was on the cottage hospitals and the community … Way back, a granny did deliveries in the isolated areas and there was no control. They weren't nurses. But between 1941 and '46, we brought in three or four at a time to the Grace Hospital for two months' training. In 1950 we had 225 trained midwives but by 1962 there were only 86 registered local midwives. We trained the last one in July of 1963. We were doing a lot of deliveries within the cottage hospitals and in the district. We didn't have the full complement of doctors or nurses in those days. We would send a nurse from the St. John's staff out to the cottage hospitals for a month or so to fill in. They didn't particularly like that, but it was the only way we could keep the hospitals going at the time. They weren't married with kids. At that time, once you got married you left nursing.

"We had to look to Britain—mainly for their midwifery. That was our main concern in those days because the nurses in the hospitals here didn't get a concentration of midwifery in their basic training. The people in the communities and the outlying areas would have been in poor shape if they hadn't had these nurses. And some of them were in areas where they hadn't had a nurse at all, so they really did make a marvelous difference. Overseas recruitment worked at the time.

"First of all there was an agency over there that we contacted. We would decide on a date that I would be going and then they would advertise, and when I got there I would know where I would be going to do the interviews. I would start off in London if there was anybody in that general area and then I went to such places as Liverpool, Bristol, Glasgow, Aberdeen, and Edinburgh, if there were applicants from those areas. Later on, we dealt through the ONA in London and they would do the advertising and the follow-up for us. They would just send me the names and addresses and I would advise the people, the date that I was interviewing, and where. I would have to make sure that there was a room available at a hotel to do the interviews.

"First of all, I looked at their qualifications because we were really concerned for the cottage hospitals and the community that they had training in midwifery. Nurses there could take specialties so if I had gone to look for someone for the Waterford Hospital, I had to make sure they had psychiatric nursing and so on.

"They usually asked questions to get a general idea of the country and the living. Some people have a pioneer spirit and it didn't bother them. The majority of the ones we recruited fit in very well. We took about a third. We had a lot of applicants, but they didn't follow through. In one place, for instance, we had six names of people who had filled in the application, but nobody turned up for their interviews. Once they got the application and you sent them a bit of information they looked at it and backtracked. I interviewed these people by myself. I had to do any follow-up too. I had a little portable typewriter with me.

"Nurses who were accepted came to St. John's first for an orientation. It depended on their background and where they were going, how long they needed to be in town. We would have the ones for cottage hospitals in St. John's for a week, and give them some of the essentials. Then we would send them out to one of the cottage hospitals to get a bit of background there before we moved them to the cottage hospital that they were really going to be working in. I can't recall anybody who had any real problems. Sometimes it took them a little while to get settled in, but once they knew people in the community, they didn't seem to have many difficulties. They signed a yearly contract. In the earlier days we might get six or seven in the run of a year; not a huge number."

The next three chapters will focus on nurses who immigrated to work on the island of Newfoundland.

Chapter One

Eastern/Central Newfoundland

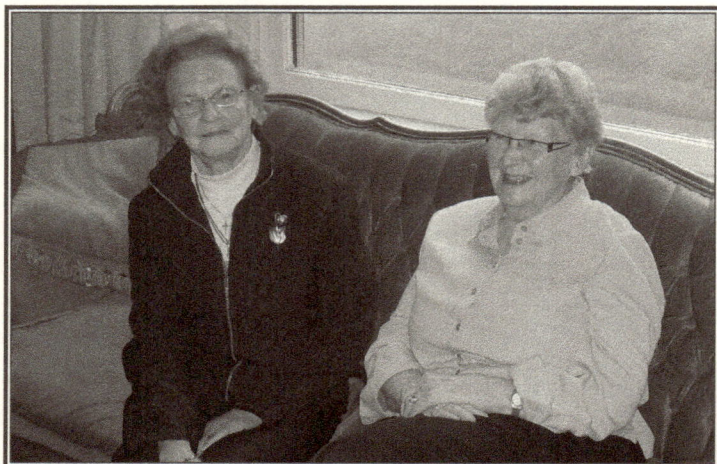

BRIGID (RICE) CHEEKS AND
ROSE (McGETTIGAN) SHEPPARD

✽

1953

"Brigid was the instigator in us coming here ... I met Brigid in London. I told her I planned to immigrate and she said she was thinking of it too and the place to go was Canada. The up and coming place was Canada."

Rose Sheppard and Brigid Cheeks immigrated to Gander together in 1953. Fifty-five years later they continue to be close friends and chose to be interviewed together.

Brigid: "We came over the year of the Queen's Coronation."

Rose: "Brigid was the instigator in us coming. I planned to go abroad but those plans were off when my friends chickened out. I was going to Australia and New Zealand, but then I met Brigid in London. I told her I planned to immigrate and she said she was thinking of it too and … the up and coming place was Canada.

"We made an application to the Overseas Nursing Service and had an interview. We had to have so many references and there were 13 people on the panel. They asked different questions about our training and what responsibilities we had. They asked if we were prepared to assist a surgeon with a caesarian section or major surgery. We both said no because we only had a short term in the OR. They insisted we take more training in the OR so we asked to withdraw our applications. Then we got a letter from Public Health in St. John's saying our qualifications were okay and to come on.

"We flew over—six hours in a propeller plane! My first impression of Gander was that it was just like the Wild West! It was an American base turned into a civilian airfield. I didn't know anything about Newfoundland before I came. I had seen it on the movies when the Queen landed at the Battery. I didn't think I made a mistake in coming because it was only for three years. We had two medicals, one before we came and another one when we got here. Jean Lewis from Public Health looked after getting our immigration papers sorted out. We had no difficulty getting registered to practice once we got here."

Brigid: "I wasn't going to come because we had only observed surgery. We didn't work in the OR. We flew into Gander. I got airsick but Rose didn't. We were here for a couple of hours then we went into St. John's for a week of orientation. We had a couple of days in St. John's and then came back to Gander on the train and had to go to work the next day. We were supposed to be trained in ether anesthesia because there was no anesthetist in Gander but nobody showed us anything. We didn't do anything in St. John's."

Rose: "I was on duty the night after we got back from St. John's but no one told me what to do. In the middle of the night, the door opened and these people came in. Nobody told me to expect people in the middle of the night and some were quite sick. We had a crash ward that was always ready for a plane crash, so I put them to bed and ordered breakfast for them. I nearly got fired! The people came on a train that ran from Clarenville to Bishop Falls. It was called the 'way freight' and the train arrived at two in the morning. They came to see the doctor and had to sit on leather chairs in the waiting room until the middle of the next day. Everything here was totally different! On the first morning that I did dressings, I used all the supplies for the month because we used forceps and absolute sterile procedure."

Brigid: "At Banting Memorial there were 30 or 40 patients. There was a male ward, a female ward, a pediatric ward, the nursery, and maternity, and we did it all. Four nurses worked there, two or three during the day, one at night and there was relief. There was an English nurse, Rose and I, and a girl from the Southern Shore. The nurses were excellent. We couldn't be made more welcome. People understood us because we spoke just like them. They pretty much spoke like Irish people."

Rose: "Shortly after we arrived I was told to go to Placentia cottage hospital as nurse-in-charge. You weren't asked, you were told! The taxi took me to Placentia and I had lunch at the Markland Hospital with the nurses. As nurse-in-charge I made up the menus and gave ether. I delivered babies, did outpatients clinic, dispensed drugs, collected the cottage hospital fees the people had to pay and kept a record of who paid. They paid in American currency and Canadian currency, and once a month the accountants came from the Department of Health. If they found a mistake I had to pay it myself. Brigid and I were trained to put screens around if we did any procedure for a patient, but in the cottage hospital you only put screens around patients when they were dying. When we put the screens around somebody all the other patients would get up and have a look.

"There were no drugstores in Placentia so I dispensed the drugs covered by the cottage hospital fees. They had big bottles of Miss

Stomach Ache and Miss Backache for your stomach and for your back. There were no drug names on these bottles. There were other medications but these two were done up in a big bottle. When the doctor was gone, I made house calls and did whatever was necessary. I had a lady with toxemia and had to deliver the baby. I did what I could do and nobody questioned me. We had a lady who was Para 10 (10 live births) from Red Island. The weather was so bad the plane couldn't land and the sea so rough they couldn't bring her in by boat. She did eventually get in but she was semi-morbid. They were hoping to save the baby, but both of them died. It was tragic! The doctor told me to tell the husband.

"The laundry for Placentia hospital was hung out on the line to dry. When the helicopters came in to land, the laundry had to be brought in so it wouldn't blow off the line. I didn't have anyone to work in the laundry and hiring was done by the Department of Health in St. John's. I called and they sent out a young girl who they said had been rehabilitated by the Salvation Army. I wasn't sure what that meant. The second night after she arrived, she went to the Argentia base with one of the nurses' aides. When they came back I was delivering a baby so I didn't see them go upstairs. I got a call from the base saying that the girls had left with their passes and they were sending over an MP to pick them up. I decided to find out what happened, and when I went to the room, the nurses' aide was in bed but obviously drunk. She didn't know where the other girl was … I couldn't find her, so I did a round of the patients. When I went into the men's ward this young girl was in bed with one of the male patients! I really got upset and the first thing I did the next morning was called St. John's and said, 'Get her out of here!'"

Brigid: "At Banting Memorial we didn't have the same responsibility as the cottage hospital because there were three doctors and always one on call. It was like a general hospital. I wasn't in the same isolation and had the supplies and supports around me. In emergency cases the helicopter would go out and get the patient."

Rose: "We were brought over by the Overseas Nursing Services and they paid our salary. The choice in Canada was Newfoundland or Winnipeg. They paid your airfare out and if you stayed three years they paid your way home. The Newfoundland government housed us in the hospital once we got here and we didn't have to pay board. Our meals were provided free and the uniform was supplied. We got a half day a week and a weekend a month."

Brigid: "I got $120 a month and Rose got $160 because she was in charge."

Rose: "Up to the time I married, I worked in general nursing, peds, and maternity, and you were expected to assist in the operating room if needed. We were jacks-of-all-trades. I thought about going back to Ireland all the time but I always liked the people in Newfoundland; that was the best part of it, the people. They've always been nice and they've always been the same. I don't regret coming over here. All my family has been here."

Brigid: "I did think about going back but I met my husband here. None of my family has been over, but I used to go home every three years."

❋

Brigid (nee Rice) Cheeks was born in Dundalk, Ireland. She graduated in 1949 as a SRN from Mayday Hospital, Surrey, England, and went on to complete midwifery (SCM), Part 1 at the Thorton Health Authority in Woking, Surrey, and Part 2 in Hackney, London, 1951. She immigrated to Banting Memorial Hospital in Gander in 1953.

Rose (nee McGettigan) Sheppard was born in Donegal, Ireland. She completed a one-year isolation (fever) nursing course in Toting, London, in 1945, graduated in 1948 as a SRN in general nursing from Mayday Hospital, Croyden, Surrey, and completed midwifery, Part I at Highgate, London, in 1950. She immigrated to work at Banting Memorial Hospital in Gander in 1953.

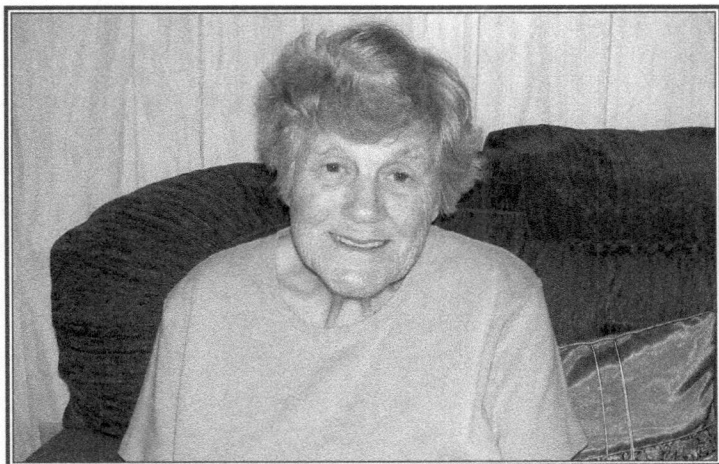

DOROTHY (BOLTON) STOCKLEY

❋

1954

*"There were 600 or 700 people there when I went there.
I was the first nurse to go there. I set up a small clinic and
ordered my own supplies, like things for dentistry and the drugs.
That came out on the coastal boat from St. John's."*

"A friend and I decided to come to Canada and there was an advertisement, by the Newfoundland government, looking for nurses. They
would pay our fare out, which was a good thing because we didn't get
paid much in those days. We had an interview with the lady who was
over recruiting for the Department of Health. I knew nothing at all
about Newfoundland before I came. We thought we were coming as
missionaries to Eskimos.

"We came on the S.S. *Nova Scotia*, which took six days. We were sick the first couple of days out but then got our sea legs. We arrived in St. John's and a lady from the Department of Health met us and took us to the Balsam Hotel. It was St. George's Day so everything was closed, and a Friday so we had the weekend to explore and see what St. John's was like. The wooden houses were a surprise to us, but we found the shops and everything interesting because we hadn't expected to find such civilization.

"We were supposed to report to the nursing service of the General Hospital at 9:00 a.m. We went to breakfast but the dining room was practically empty. After breakfast we walked over to the place, and lo and behold the time had gone back the night before so it was 10:00 when we got there! We were on our copybooks right away! We had two weeks' orientation in St. John's. We had to learn the names of the drugs because medications here were different. We had a day with a dentist learning how to pull teeth. Then we learned by experience—trial and error! We went with a district nurse to different places in St. John's. Then I was sent to Springdale for orientation to the hospital there. I worked there for a month, came back to St. John's for more orientation, then went to Lamaline to work with the district nurse there. That was a learning experience because I hadn't done any district nursing, only district midwifery. I went everywhere with the nurse on her visits and watched what she did. I didn't have difficulty understanding the people. Some of the language was different, but most people spoke regular English. Then I was stationed in Greenspond, Bonavista Bay, as a district nurse. I went to Greenspond and my friend went to Burgeo hospital.

"I went by train from St. John's to Gambo, then by boat from Gambo. The Anglican minister met me. He was in charge of the nursing committee and arranged to get a nurse in Greenspond, which is an island about three miles in circumference. There were 600 or 700 people there when I went there. I was the first nurse to go there. I set up a small clinic and ordered my own supplies, like things for dentistry and the drugs. That came out on the coastal boat from St. John's.

"I was accepted very well by the people in Greenspond. I did home and school visits in the morning. We had three schools: Salvation Army, United Church and Anglican. The home visits were mainly postnatal care or if anybody asked me to visit. I did dressings in the home and sometimes I just diagnosed, because people didn't know what was wrong with them. I did quite a lot of prenatal work and home deliveries. The doctor was at Brookfield hospital, which was a cottage hospital about half an hour by boat. He never visited unless I sent for him. There was no telephone in those days, only ship-to-shore, but I didn't worry about being on my own because when you're young, you think you can do anything.

"I had clinic hours from two to four in the afternoon. Then if there was another visit I had to make, I did it before I went home. The clinic was for people with colds, with cuts that needed stitching or needed a tooth pulled. The people went to the hospital for a lot of things, but if the doctor in Brookfield said they needed a dressing or something, they came to the clinic. Also there was no pharmacy, so they got their medicines from the hospital or the clinic. Everything was paid by the government but the people paid for extractions; 50 cents a tooth.

"I remember one girl who hemorrhaged after she delivered. I phoned for the doctor and a helicopter to come for her. She had a cervical tear. There was a man on the island who knew his blood type was O Positive, so we took blood from him and gave it to her before they moved her. She survived and the baby was okay. Unfortunately, she was negative and she had two other babies after that and had to go into St. John's for antibodies. I had another lady who started having seizures after her baby was born. We took her to hospital by boat, but unfortunately she died.

"When they pluck the feathers off sea birds, they have boiling water in the tub. This little fellow was walking backwards and fell into the tub and scalded his back. I soaked a sheet in bicarbonate soda and wrapped him in it. We took him to the hospital by boat because it was quicker than waiting for the helicopter from Gander, but he died shortly afterwards from kidney failure.

"I had a 12-year-old girl who I knew had appendicitis, but couldn't get her off the island for three days. I was anxious about her but we kept ice packs on her appendix area and managed to get her over to hospital in time. She survived.

"Shortly after I went to Greenspond I had a crib death. I had to write the death certificate, so I phoned the doctor. I said, 'I don't know what happened to this baby.' He said, 'Put down crib death.' He diagnosed it from across the ocean!

"I had a little boy who was playing a game called Pippy where they hit a stick. It hit his eye. When I looked at it I knew he had lost his eye because the vitreous humor was leaking out. We got him to the hospital but he lost the sight in the eye.

"I was in Greenspond for 13 years. I got married and had six children, but my husband had been married before and had six older children. We had quite a family! I left because my children were growing up and I figured they'd get a better education in Gander. Also I wanted to get into a hospital setting because the responsibility of the district was getting a little much for me.

"I've been back to England for visits. My family didn't visit when I was in Greenspond, but my sister has been over several times since I came to Gander. I'm happy I came to Newfoundland. I wouldn't go back to England now."

❋

Dorothy Amy (nee Bolton) Stockley was born in Broadstairs, Kent, England. She completed her SRN at the University College Hospital in London, England, in 1951. In 1954 she completed midwifery at Margate, Kent, before immigrating as the first nurse to work in Greenspond, Bonavista Bay.

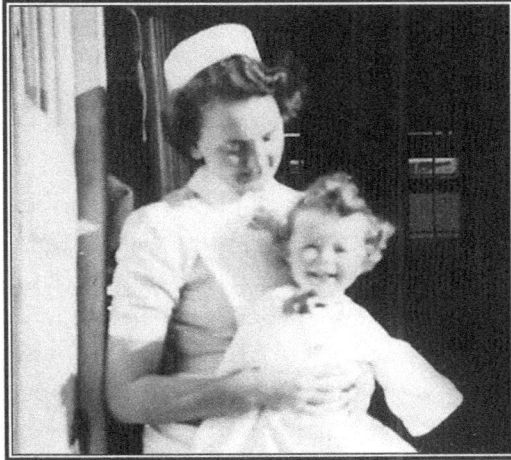

BARBARA (TRENT) MOULTON

❋

1957

*"A nice girl who was all bright and breezy met us from the
Department of Health and said, 'Are you staying for one year? I hope
you are staying for two years.' I said, 'No we are not! We'll stay for one.'
I was just tired by that time! And now 50 years later, here I am!"*

"A friend and I both liked travelling and had decided to go somewhere
but didn't know where. We made inquiries and decided on Newfoundland. The idea was that we would work here for a year, then work
our way across Canada, but I didn't get off the island! Neither of us did.
I met my husband, got married and had children.

"I came in October of 1957. We weren't recruited. We saw an
advertisement and followed it up. We tried to find out something about

Newfoundland but didn't find out very much. It sounded interesting so we decided to come. I was interviewed by Jean Lewis in London. I didn't have any problems getting licensed. Apart from getting a passport and having a medical done, we didn't really have to do any of the preparation.

"We flew here and at that time, planes were Turbo Props. We were two and a half hours out over the Atlantic when one of the engines gave out and we had to fly back to London. We transferred to another plane and left again. Before we got to Gander we were told we weren't going to land there and were going on to Sydney. We sat in Sydney airport all day and finally they got us a flight into St. John's. We got here sometime that night. I phoned the Department of Health and they sent someone to meet us …. It was an auspicious beginning! A nice girl, who was bright and breezy met us from the Department of Health and said, 'Are you staying for one year? I hope you are staying for two years.' I said, 'No we are not! We'll stay for one.' I was just tired by that time! And now 50 years later, here I am!

"We had a three-day orientation in St. John's. We asked to be posted together, but we were told I was going to Burin and my friend Beryl was going to Bonavista. When I said to the interviewer that I thought we were going to be posted together, she said, 'You can spend the weekend at Goobies.' When we drove through there I thought 'A weekend here?' It was the end of October so it was dark for most of the trip. We were in a taxi with other people and it took a good eight hours to get there. From Goobies on we dropped people off in the middle of nowhere. There were no lights to be seen and people would say, 'Somebody is picking me up here in a boat.' We finally got to Burin and as we drove by the cliffs, some men were using a rope to pull a car that had gone over the cliffs. I discovered later that they were hospital staff in the car.

"Burin cottage hospital was built with funding from a lottery. Al Capone was supposed to be involved because people said he spent a lot of time in St. Pierre. It was an old 50-bed hospital with the basics but quite a switch from St. Thomas. I used to think, 'If St. Thomas could see me now!' There were three other nurses and one doctor when I went there, but over a period of time, two nurses left, and for a long time there were just two of us and one doctor.

"We agreed not to take weekends off and to do call every second night because somebody had to be there. I didn't get too many weekends off to spend in Goobies! There were no set hours, you just worked. When there were things to be done, you had to do them. Basically we worked from 8:00 'til 5:00, then whoever was on call that night went off at 5:00, because invariably the maternity cases were in the middle of the night. We had untrained aides and maids. On top of everything else, we had to train them on the job and there wasn't much time for that. Some were excellent and we relied on them, particularly for maternity cases.

"We got paid more than we got in England because the pay was pitiful over there. We worked hard and didn't have regular hours. Periodically we got another nurse and then there were three of us, which was much better. Sometimes, if two labour cases came in, you'd have to get up on the night that you weren't on call because nurses handled all the labour and delivery. We did … a lot of midwifery work, but if we ran into any complications we called the doctor.

"In the 15 months I worked in Burin I delivered 88 babies, and I wasn't the only one delivering babies. Everyone had big families in those days. There was another English girl who came a month before I did and two Newfoundland nurses. They received me very well and I didn't have any problems. The only trouble we had was the aides didn't understand us. We were both English but the other girl had a Northern England accent which was different from mine. I'd be in one room and she'd be in another room and one of the aides would say, 'Ms. Trent, what did Ms. Monue just tell me?' I'd say, 'I don't know. I wasn't there!' It was funny! Then they would ask her what I said. But they were good, very willing, and we relied on each other because we had to.

"We had a five-year-old boy admitted with pneumonia, who developed chicken pox while he was in and was smothered in spots. We had a coal furnace and the janitor kept the place boiling hot. I was asleep one night and about three o'clock an aide came up and said, 'Miss Trent, could you come down? Meryl won't go to sleep and he won't stay in bed.' I went down and he was so itchy he was going crazy. I got calamine lotion and sponged him down. Then I took the blankets off and put a sheet over him. I said, 'Meryl, I won't put the blanket on because you'll get too hot and itch again.' He looked at me and said, 'And if ya gets cold, ya dies.' I said, 'Have the blanket!'

"At first I did have difficulty understanding the locals even when taking their names in clinic. They would say, 'Katen.' And I would say, 'How do you spell that?' and they would spell Keating. Then they had 'some wonderful pain' or 'wonderful hemorrhage.' One nurse told me of an old lady who came with her husband who had died very suddenly of a stroke or an aneurism. The woman said, 'He was sittin' der and all of a sudden he swallied and glutched and he died.' Then there was 'Yes, b'y,' whether it was a man or woman; I'd think, 'I'm not a boy!' Also it was difficult knowing what they meant sometimes. Things like 'I finds me back' or 'I finds me knee' didn't give you any hint that there was pain.

"One night we had a pregnant lady come in who was very toxic. The doctor had just graduated and come from Ireland. He decided to do a section although he had never done one, only assisted. I scrubbed. We had an anesthetic machine but we weren't allowed to use it—not that we knew how to use it! The other nurse had to give the anesthetic, which was just dripping ether onto a mask. She was sitting at the head of the table dripping the ether onto the mask and not having done it before, she didn't realize she was leaning over it. All of a sudden she collapsed! She didn't slide right off the stool, but we had to grab everything and hang on until she came around. The baby and mother were fine but somebody must have been looking out for us that night.

"I had an old fisherman come to the clinic one night. I was putting screens around him and thought he said, 'I've got boils.' So I said, 'Do you have many?' and he said, 'No.' When I asked where they were, he was red in the face. I said, 'Are they down the back of your neck or under your arms?' He said, 'I said I got piles.' I'm sure he was thinking, 'Who is this bright English nurse asking where they are?'

"We dispensed drugs. The doctor didn't keep a record, only the notes in his chart, so we would go into what we called the pharmacy and find a pill that matched the one the patient brought in with them. They always brought some in. But I didn't give many drugs without a doctor and especially not to children. I didn't take any chances. With an adult you get a good idea, but anything that I couldn't handle with children, I called the doctor. I had a maternity case where the baby's heart rate was dropping and there were signs that the baby was in distress. I found the doctor on call, told him what was going on and said, 'You need to come and give me some advice.' He just said, 'You've handled it quite well, so I won't bother. Let me know if you have any more problems.' But everything turned out all right.

"I delivered the 18th baby of a local woman. Then a year or so after I was married and was expecting my first child, I met this woman in the hospital. She said to me, 'I don't suppose you remember me. You delivered my 18th baby.' I said I remembered her, then asked, 'I don't suppose you've had any further children?' She said, 'I had a twin since then.' She was a very soft-spoken woman and sort of slow in her speech and there was a long pause before she said, 'But I don't think I wants any more.' I thought that was so funny!

"The people in the community were very supportive of me, which surprised me when you think how little Britain did for Newfoundland. One older lady who was so loyal to the British nurses would say, 'There was nothing like a British nurse. They did more than anybody.' The people were kind. You got a few rough ones but not very many.

"It took time adjusting to Burin having come from London. I've always been open to new experiences and always had a sense of humour. I missed the spring and music. I always liked classical music, but all there was at that time was Kitty Wells and country music. There was no theatre. Even in church, the hymns were desperately slow. The weather wasn't easy. It was dirt roads from St. John's to Burin and I first came in for a break in January. We got stuck in St. John's because the roads were blocked and muddy. It wasn't snow but mud. I didn't get another break until August when we got two weeks holidays. My friend and I didn't know what we were going to do but we came into St. John's. We got the train here and went to Corner Brook. We stayed at the Simms Hotel and people were very friendly. They drove us around and showed us the place. Somebody said the Northern Ranger was in and that we might enjoy that. So we got on in Corner Brook and went back to St. John's. We got two weeks holidays. Other than that I stayed in Burin.

"I came for a year then met my husband nine months after I got here. They had line dances but I hadn't been to one. I knew a couple of nurses who wanted me to come to the lines time and I thought, 'Why not?' I went; my husband was there and that was the beginning of it. I discovered afterwards that several people had decided I would be a good wife for my husband and arranged for us both to be at this dance. He didn't know it and I didn't know it. Anyway, it worked! That was September; we got engaged in December and were married in January. I didn't work after I married, but at the time there weren't a lot of married women who worked and we wanted children right away. Also, my husband was of the generation where his wife didn't work. I wanted my family to meet my husband and vice versa so we went home the next year."

❋

Barbara (nee Trent) Moulton was born in Devonshire, England. She completed two years in children's orthopedics at the Mayor Treloar

Orthopaedic Hospital in Alton, Hampshire, in 1951 before going on to obtain her SRN in 1954 from Nightingale Training School, St. Thomas's Hospital in London. She completed midwifery Part 1 at St. Mary's in Manchester and Part 2 at County Hospital in Dorchester in 1955. She immigrated in 1957 to work at Burin cottage hospital.

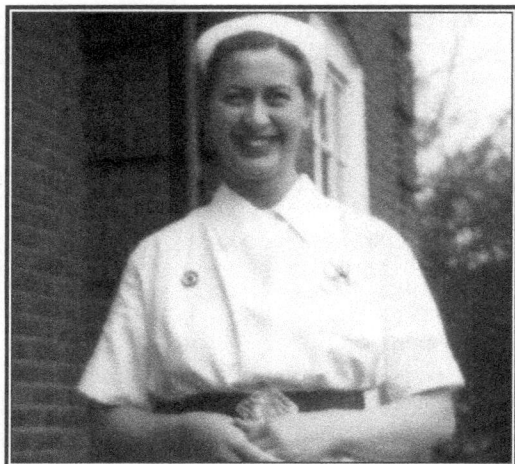

PAULA (BALLANTINE) McDONALD

❀

1962

"It was just a relaxed, comfortable welcome. They had put in supplies and coal and wood in the fireplace. It was as if family had prepared it for us. It was a lovely house. I looked out the upstairs and thought, 'My heavens, we are really meant to be here!'"

"Malcolm went to the British Medical Association House in London to find out about the prospects in Canada. The gentleman there said, 'There is somebody here from Newfoundland. Maybe you would like to speak with him?' Later Malcolm told me that the doctor he met painted a glorious picture of Newfoundland. It was like the Bahamas of the North Atlantic. So we decided that we wanted to be in Newfoundland.

"We had a pet otter, Pooh, and it was the reason we moved. My husband got in touch with Dr. Collingwood and said, 'We've got this pet otter and we've decided to bring her. Is that all right?' 'Yes,' he said, 'of course there is no problem there.' He found out that all that was required was that she'd come in a clean travelling box with no straw. We came on the Trans Canada Airlines in December 1962. When we arrived it was very mild.

"We were in St. John's at the Newfoundland Hotel for 10 days. The hotel's manager and his children would come and watch the otter play in the bath. It was fun and everybody was adorable to us. Most of our dealings were with the Department of Health related to Malcolm's work.

"Our drive to Bonavista was dramatic. There had been what I thought was an enormous snowfall but now, 40 years later, I realize it wasn't too bad at all! A forest fire had left mile upon mile of awful devastation, with black stumps sticking up through the snow. It was really morbid; it was a horrible, desolate, dreadful feeling. We got to Brookfield and had the loveliest welcome from the head nurse, Ben Winsor. They were so friendly and nice to us. It was just a relaxed, comfortable welcome. They had put in supplies and coal and wood in the fireplace. It was as if family had prepared it for us. It was a lovely house. I looked out the upstairs and thought, 'My heavens, we are really meant to be here!'

"I didn't work as a nurse. An otter takes up a lot of time, and Malcolm and I didn't feel it was appropriate for me to be in the work team. I wanted nothing to do with the politics of the hospital and I thought the nurses might feel uncomfortable with the doctor's wife. As friends, we just got on like a house on fire. We came to an arrangement where I lit the fire and I told them, 'When you see the smoke, tea is on.' They were welcome to come over and we'd have toast and cheese, a bit of cake or a biscuit. It was women getting together and we'd discuss things they were involved in, problems they faced, and experiences they had. Sometimes they were terribly busy.

"I felt very welcome in the community. Eric and June Winter's store was across the road and he was the first one to come over. He was a lovely man and June was adorable. We played cards with them a lot and sometimes the nurses would join us. We also used to make wine. Another couple we got to know was Skipper Tom Blackwood and his wife, who were great berry pickers and great with nautical terms. You never 'went in the car'; you 'got aboard the car.' If you went over a difficult path you 'went aground.' We got a huge kick out of it. Once Malcolm went to visit him and whichever way he turned the car, it wasn't to the skipper's liking. 'Doctor, boy,' he said, 'you've done that all wrong. You should have rolled in the heave and slewed us down around. You're doing too much driving!'

"We socialized with the community. They would come for a 'time.' Suddenly we'd hear footsteps with no warning. But they came prepared. In lobster season we had our supply of liquid refreshment and they came with the lobsters. The ladies brought bread and cookies. Then we sat in the kitchen having the greatest feed. We had a ball.

"Mabel Norris was head nurse in Brookfield and very early on I decided I would do a devilled chicken. Mabel came over and I said, 'If you want a cup of tea you have to make it yourself because I'm doing devilled chicken.' I mixed up the ingredients and smeared the yellowy brown mixture over the chicken then put it to marinate. It must have looked pretty horrible. Then she came back when it was cooking and said, 'That smells good! I'm not going until I've had some.' So I said, 'Stay for supper.' And she had devilled chicken from then on. Introducing curry was another thing.

"Somebody gave Malcolm a saltwater duck which was cleaned, and I asked the man how to cook it. He said, 'The same way as you cook a chicken.' I put onion dressing in and stuck it in the oven, but I thought it smelled a bit fishy. Malcolm came home and said, 'Paula, whatever it is, bury it!' The nurses knew how to cook duck so we exchanged the tricks of the trade. We had plenty of cooking sessions.

"My first Easter here, there was a knock on the door. Snow was falling and two little chaps about eight were at the door. They said, 'Do you want to buy an Easter card?' I thought it strange because I never sent anybody an Easter Card in my life. I said, 'Come in. What are you doing out this hour of the night in a raging storm?' It wasn't really raging, but to me it was, and I thought it was irresponsible of the parents to allow them out. Then I realized, 'Their parents don't know they were out selling Easter cards and would probably get a fright.' So I decided they were going to stay until Malcolm could take them home. I took their coats, asked if they'd like hot chocolate. I had chocolate-covered cookies for the minister in case he came to visit. I put them on a tray and when I looked there wasn't a biscuit left. Their little cheeks were bulging! They had stuffed their mouths full! I was afraid they would choke, so I said, 'Spit those out and eat them one at a time or you'll choke!' They went into gales of laughter, not knowing what to make of me. I asked, 'Do you have any brothers and sisters?' and 'Where do you go to school?' the usual questions. When I ran out of questions, one of them announced, 'Uncle Harry Andrews' toilet took off.' I said, 'Took off? Where did it take off to?' He put his arm in the great gesture of clear across the bay, so I said, 'Good God! He wasn't in it was he?' It was an outhouse on the edge of the cliff and it had taken off in the wind. I never heard anything so funny in my life. I just loved them!

"The children in the community loved the otter. A little girl, Charity Blackwood, would bring her dog, Timmy. I would take Paddy, our dog, and Pooh, and we would go for walks, then come back and look through the Eaton's catalogue. I got into the lifestyle very quickly.

"We were in Bonavista for four years. Pooh died of a thiamine deficiency because smelt contains thiamine-destroying factor and she ate a lot of smelts. I never worked there. I had too much fun. I learned to bake bread and I visited people that Malcolm was concerned about. I'd go on a social visit but then do an assessment so they weren't alarmed. It was all very informal and easy going.

"Then in April '67 we came to St. John's. I went to see Janet Story who was the director of nurses and did a refresher course with Mrs. Ash. After that, I worked with people with aneurisms and spinal fusions.

"I regard Newfoundland as home. I have more friends here than in Britain. I love it here and feel this is where I belong."

❊

Frances Paula (nee Ballantine) McDonald was born in Banglore, India. She graduated from the Hove General and Royal Sussex County Hospital in Brighton, England, in 1952 as a SRN. She immigrated in 1962 with her husband, who was a physician recruited for Bonavista cottage hospital.

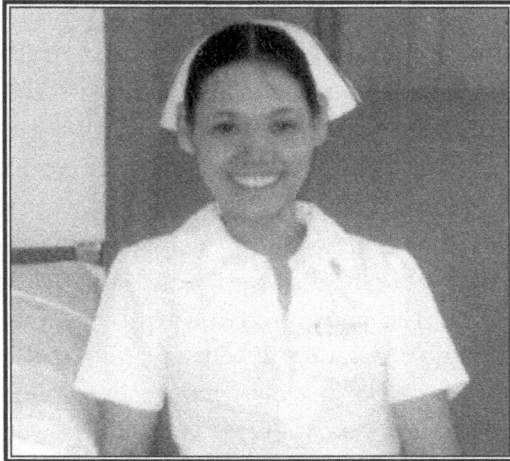

DELIAH (DOMINGUEZ) GUY

❋

1974

*"Having so many people from my culture in Twillingate
helped eased the transition. People opened their arms to us and
I didn't have much problem adapting. The two things that
challenged me were the weather and the food."*

"I decided to come to Canada because I thought it was a peaceful place
to live and that people were friendly. Newfoundland was the first job
opportunity given to me so I said, 'I don't care what part of Canada it
is as long as I got the job.' Mrs. White was the Director of Nursing in
Twillingate. I communicated with her and did the contract for my job
placement. I signed the job contract by special delivery. And the rest is
history!

"Getting to Twillingate was an experience. On my way to there I ended up at the wrong airport. I came to St. John's because my ticket said St. John's, Newfoundland, but I was supposed to be at Gander. I had faith in the travel agent when she said, 'Don't worry about anything. All you have to do is relax. Somebody will pick you up.' I thought, 'That's easy.' When I told people I was going, they cried to break their hearts because this was my first time away from home and the first time on a plane. Mom didn't want me to go, but I said, 'Mom, I have to go. We have to sacrifice. The only way I can help you financially is to do this.' At home, nursing was very expensive and my school of nursing was very exclusive. Some of my classmates were the daughters of the governor and millionaires but we were not rich. We were not poor. We ate three times a day but we were barely making it.

"Before I left the Philippines, my mom said, 'You don't have to worry about anything because somebody is always looking after you. That is the one up there. You'll be fine.' Then I get off the plane and I'm in the wrong airport! I didn't know the difference in Gander and St. John's. I was scared to death! I'm in a foreign land! I hadn't eaten in three days because I didn't eat on the plane. They had salad in the plane, but I couldn't eat that because that was only for animals. I only had fruit and lost eight pounds in three days because I wasn't used to the food. At home we ate rice seven days a week, two to five times a day.

"A man at the airport knew I was scared to ask for help. Because Mom had said, 'Don't trust anybody because you don't know what will happen.' That stuck in my head. But this one man kept looking at me and it scared me to death. I was a foreigner. Anyway, the man approached me because my luggage was going around and around. It was about a 150 pounds and I couldn't lift it. He said, 'Did you come from the Philippines? You look frightened but don't worry; I married a girl from the Philippines.' I started crying and it struck me that Mom was right. It was my destiny to meet these people and a woman who had worked in Twillingate. They asked me to stay the night. It was

44

March and I was wearing a blazer and high-heeled shoes. I think of ice as the ice in a drink, but here I was stepping on ice. I couldn't believe it! When I met the woman, she gave me a beautiful coat, which is something I will never forget. In the morning it was beautiful and they took me to the airport and said, 'Don't worry. Somebody will pick you up and everything will be fine.' I said to myself, 'Here we go again!' But they were right because someone was waiting for people going to Twillingate.

"The flight from St. John's to Gander cost $27.50 and I only had $30.00. I talked to Mrs. White but had to pay for that because it wasn't part of the contract. To go from Gander to Twillingate cost $40.00, but that was covered by the hospital. I was frightened to death because I was in a vehicle with a male I didn't know, and it was just the two of us going from Gander to Twillingate. He didn't talk to me and I had my rosary beads. He must have heard because I was saying to myself, 'Oh my God. Is this the right place? How come there are not many houses? How come the houses are so tiny?' I was scared to death! About a half-hour before Twillingate he started to talk and I felt a bit better. When we got to Twillingate, he said, 'That's the nurses' residence where you're staying. The hospital is the small building.' I thought, 'My God, where am I going?' I couldn't believe it was the hospital.

"When I came there were 23 Filipino nurses in Twillingate. I got to know the areas of the Philippines they came from. Our main language is Tagalog, and Spanish is the second language. I speak a bit of Spanish but some of the Filipino nurses didn't speak the same dialect. I felt bad because they spoke Tagalog, but I didn't understand it. We had developed a friendly relationship and it was like a community. There were only three Canadian nurses in Twillingate when I went there. It was a challenge to be in a place where everybody knows everybody and everybody speaks to you. There was no discrimination. They treated us like their own and were very friendly. The challenge I had in Twillingate was how the people speak. We spoke English fluently because our education is based on American and English books. We were taught the right English.

"Two questions we asked after a patient's morning care were 'Have you peed?' and 'Have you pooped?' These were slang words to me. I had an 85-year-old man who was a little hard of hearing. I took his temperature and blood pressure and asked him, 'Have you defecated? Have you urinated?' He said, 'What, nurse?' I asked him again, but he didn't understand what I was talking about. By now I'm getting uncomfortable and he is getting upset. One of the LPNs asked me if I was having a problem with him and I said, 'He doesn't understand what I'm talking about.' She said to him, 'What was the last time you peed?' 'This morning,' he said. I had to get the swing of it because they have a different terminology and they speak so fast in Twillingate. Now I understand it all and they consider me a Newfie because of the way I talk. I still have my accent, but I don't think you can take that away from me.

"Having so many people from my culture in Twillingate helped ease the transition. People opened their arms to us and I didn't have much problem adapting. The two things that challenged me were the weather and the food. Today I'd rather be cold than hot because if you're cold you can put things on. Food was another thing but I adjusted to it very well. Now it doesn't bother me. I think I adjusted in about two or three months, but the hardest part was missing Mom, Dad and the family. I'm not a happy-go-lucky person, but I think being able to adapt to any situation is important.

"I worked in Twillingate from 1974 to '78 and was the head nurse when I left. I never regretted going to Twillingate because that was where my experience came from. It was a rural hospital and I delivered more than 100 babies; four were named after me. All the Filipino nurses delivered babies in Twillingate then, especially if the doctors were having their sleep. The doctors would ask who was on duty and when you'd say who it was, they'd say, 'I'll have a good night and won't be woken up.' I delivered babies feet first and shoulder first, which was challenging. But it was amazing, the experience we were given and the privilege to do for the patients. Being a nurse in that kind of rural setting is challenging yet satisfying.

"I will never forget Twillingate. I fell in love with the place and it was my second home. I worked with an LPN who looked out for us all the time. I met my husband at a little staff party but I was with somebody else. We met again after a year and that was it. It was meant to be.

"I settled in Gander but my second home is Twillingate. That is where my heart is and I fell in love with the place. I was back to the Philippines in 1987 with my husband and my son for my parents' 50th wedding anniversary, but I don't think I will ever live anywhere except here in Newfoundland."

❀

Delilah (nee Dominguez) Guy born in Sineguelasan, Bacoor, Cavite, Philippines. She graduated in 1971 from San Juan De Dios Hospital in Manila with a Bachelor of Nursing and worked there for a couple of years. She immigrated to work at the hospital in Twillingate in 1974.

VALERIE TWEEDIE

❀

1975

"We came as landed immigrants ...
and I got more points than he did. They wanted
the nurses. The vet was quite by the by!
So I swung the immigration."

"We came to Newfoundland because of my uncle. My husband is an avid salmon fisherman. My uncle, who was in the Merchant Navy, told him about Newfoundland and salmon fishing. There was an advert in the Veterinary Record looking for a vet to join a practice in Grand Falls. My husband applied, never thinking anybody would even phone him, let alone turn up and interview him. The vet in question came to England and did an interview. My husband came the end of March. I came in April. I got rid of all our stuff in Britain. We didn't intend to stay. We came for an adventure and something different and to decide what we'd do from there. Thirty-two years later we're still here!

"We came as landed immigrants and the process took us about six months. We were awarded points to immigrate and I got more points than he did but they wanted nurses. The vet was quite by-the-by! I swung the immigration! We chuckled about that because they didn't deny he was needed; I just got more points as a nurse.

"I had done a degree program and I had more than the standard amount of midwifery, although I didn't do the midwifery certificate. I also had a lot more than the standard amount of psychiatry so I didn't have to write exams to register. I contacted the hospital in Grand Falls before I left Britain and went for an interview when I got here and started work about 10 days after arriving. That was a bit of a shock! When I came, the health care system was very different. I came from a large teaching hospital to what I felt was a bit of a backwater. The hospital was a fair size, but not what I was used to, as a teaching hospital has a different atmosphere completely. Grand Falls had the nursing assistant program so there were educators about but it was quite different. The nurses even had different roles. They were doing a lot of things we weren't doing in Britain. Nurses were dealing with lab results, notifying doctors, just more hands-on, whereas in Britain that wasn't part of our role.

"The orientation didn't stump me because I had done a lot of it, where we had done a degree. I didn't request anything in particular so there was an opening on medicine and I got put there. It was quite a difficult floor. I discovered afterward that nobody wanted to work there, but it didn't bother me because I like medical nursing.

"Some of the medications were called by the trade names, which was different. One thing that hit me was the use of narcotics or rather the lack of use of narcotics might be more appropriate. We had a lot of terminal patients on the medical floor and one patient was not well controlled with his pain medication. I remember saying, 'Why don't you use dimorphine?' They looked at me and said, 'What's that?' I said, 'Heroine.' They were horrified. I had administered it in Britain and knew how well it worked. I remember thinking, 'Oh dear, I stuck my foot in it again!' I was good at sticking my foot in it quite inadvertently.

"I found things here quite different, but I think it was the way that floor was run. I didn't like it and felt it could be run better. They wanted things done the way they had always done it. Under the old system everybody was allocated tasks. One nursing assistant got assigned blood pressures; another assigned to giving drinks and I found that strange. To me, you shouldn't have to be told to give a patient a drink of water. The head nurse went on holiday for a month after I had been there for about four months. We had such a high turnover in staff that I had shot up in seniority and I found myself in charge. I changed things while she was gone, but I didn't do it all on my own. It was simple things like assigning patients so they did all the care for that patient. We tried it and the nursing assistants loved it and they backed me up when the head nurse came back. We kept that system.

"I don't know if I was accepted by the nurses in Grand Falls. I think I was a bit of a novelty, my accent for a start. I had trouble with certain words and I would ask for things that were named differently. The patients would say, 'I haven't got a clue what you said, but I could listen to you all day!' There were a number of non-Canadian nurses. There was fair number of Filipinos and they did tend to stick together. There was also a number of Indians.

"I was there three weeks when I had to give a talk on terminal care because the head nurse wouldn't do it. It was a bit alarming because I hadn't done anything like that, but it was something I thought was very important. Had I stayed in Scotland I probably would have ended up in palliative care. Part of me didn't mind doing it but part of me was very nervous. There were an awful lot of other people there that weren't nursing assistants, so I don't know if they decided they wanted to hear what she has to say, or if it was curiosity. I think I was a bit of a novelty. I was 22, just moved to a new country, and just married. It was a bit nerve-wracking.

"I tried to do the coronary care program that fall. Coronary care had always appealed to me. The program was offered a couple of evenings a week but I had to drop it because I couldn't get enough cooperation to change my shifts when I needed to. I found that very disconcerting because I was trying to do something to improve myself but not getting the cooperation or support. I did eventually do it when we moved to Gander in 1981.

"We were in Grand Falls for five years. I had a child in 1976 so I worked for a year and a bit full-time, and after he was born I went back on a casual basis. I never went back full-time. I am a little bit old-fashioned that way."

"When we came to Gander I continued to work casual. It was a completely different hospital. I found it much better. I worked until about 1990, but I was also doing the veterinary business. I was raising three sons with a husband who was on the road a good part of the time and I couldn't cope with it all.

"The one thing I missed was the camaraderie. I felt part of the nursing, as much as you can when you work casual. My career was short but it was interesting and it was what I wanted."

❋

Valerie Tweedie was born in Edinburgh, Scotland. She graduated with a Bachelor of Social Science in Nursing from Edinburgh University in 1975 and as a RGN. She completed a District Nursing Certificate in 1975 before immigrating with her husband, who was recruited to Grand Falls as a vet in 1975.

Chapter Two

WESTERN NEWFOUNDLAND

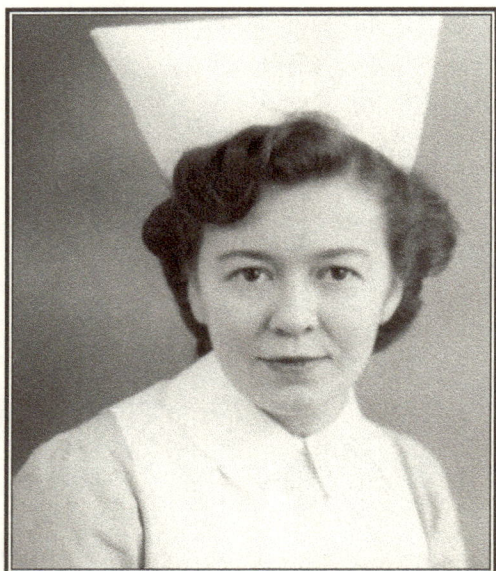

DOREEN (JANES) ROSS

❀

1954

*"When we arrived in Ramea … The first day we were going out,
Ruby said to me, 'Don't forget to put on your smile because
everyone will be peeking from behind the curtains to see what the
new nurse is like.' I felt like a Cheshire cat …."*

"I noticed a tiny advertisement in a nursing magazine for Newfoundland for cottage hospital and district. I wrote out of curiosity because having done three qualifications I thought, 'Enough of that, time I got to work!' I received a letter that I had an appointment at the Waverley

Hotel with Jean Lewis. She had the map of Newfoundland and talked about what it was like, the isolation, and really sold the outports to me. I was fascinated and it was a challenge.

"I arrived in Gander and was put in a room at the Saturn Hotel. To my horror, I was put with another person, luckily a female. The following morning I flew to St. John's and was met at the airport by an English nurse from the Department of Health. I asked how long she'd been here. When she said, 'Five years,' I thought, 'That's a lifetime!'

"I stayed at a house on Cochrane Street where students from the outports stayed. That evening Jean Lewis came while we were having supper and gave me my ticket to fly out the next day. When I went back everyone asked where I was going. I said, 'I didn't catch it, something Crossing.' The comment around the table was 'Don't tell her; let her find out.' It was Stephenville Crossing. I was there six weeks for orientation because cottage hospitals were constantly short of staff.

"There were four nurses there, myself included. In my first week, Dr. Dermot Murphy asked if I'd ever given an anesthetic. I said, 'Just chloroform for obstetrics.' He said, 'You can give your first one under my direction. I'm doing an appendectomy.' That was my first anesthetic and the patient survived! The medical assistant there showed me how to pull teeth and I remember he broke each one off, which I never did. It was nothing to find in the morning a patient on the OR table and one on the x-ray table. We were that short of bed space. We put newborn babies in a drawer and I've seen four newborn babies side by side in a crib. You had to use the facilities you had! I came for a challenge and I got it! The only thing I missed were flowers on visiting day. You saw very few flowers around Stephenville Crossing.

"One day a Mountie came to check on a man who was hired to escort a patient to the mental hospital. The Mountie asked how things were going and I said, 'Fine.' The next thing I knew he was dragging the man along the corridor and the Mountie had one arm in a cast! The women on the ward were looking out the window as the Mountie bumped this sitter down the front steps of the hospital. He was drinking and that wasn't allowed! I just couldn't believe what I was seeing. Talk about the Wild West!

"I came to St. John's for a month of orientation and did visits with public health and child welfare nurses. I was sent to Garnish for one week with an elderly English nurse who had been there many years. She showed me how to do things in the district. My recollection was popping into houses, being shown the beautiful handiwork they did, and checking a blood pressure here and there.

"Then I was shipped off to Ramea because I had applied to go to a district. Ruby Harnett came with me from the department. She stayed a few days, then I was on my own. We were 26 hours crossing by train to Port Aux Basques. We went into the dining room for dinner and Ruby said, 'Dr. Spurrell has replaced Dr. Gough in Burgeo and I don't know how the charge nurse is getting on with him.' I hadn't a clue who these people were! A lady with a little girl about two was sitting opposite us, and Ruby put a spoon into a napkin to make a doll. She noticed the woman had a Grace ring and spoke to her. Who should it be but Dr. Spurrell's wife travelling back!

"We got the boat from Port Aux Basques to Burgeo and a steamer to Ramea. We had to wait for the steamer, which carried freight down the coast. It was my lifeline with the outside world! I got mail when the boat went down from Port Aux Basques one week and had to have my mail ready when the boat came up the next week.

"When we arrived in Ramea there were two ladies in labour. Ruby and I ran from one to the other with a huge maternity bag and both children arrived safely. The first day we visited, Ruby said, 'Don't forget to smile because everyone will be peeking from behind the curtains to see what the new nurse is like.' I felt like a Cheshire cat going around.

"Canon Honeygold, the Anglican minister in Burgeo, said there was to be a meeting and Ruby said to me, 'You're going to have to speak to the people.' They wanted to meet the new nurse but I got through that. Afterwards we were invited to the welfare officer's house and offered a drink. I didn't drink but being polite, I agreed. Ruby just sat there while I took a sip and when she saw my face, she said, 'I'm sure they won't mind if you don't drink it!' On the south coast it was common for people to have alcohol from St. Pierre—and I mean alcohol! Evidently they diluted it with juice.

"A friend and I went to dinner at Maloney's, and walking back I saw a light on an island where nobody had lived for years. I asked what the light was and he said, 'They're either burying or digging it up.' The people buried liquor on the island to hide it from the Mounties. I remember thinking, 'We're back in Dickens' time!' There was a wooden bungalow behind Maloney's house and if anyone wanted a bottle, the man there sold it. Rum was very much a Newfoundland drink. For me it was a naval drink and I never thought women drank it! There was also whiskey and cherry brandy. They went in dories to St. Pierre and brought back five-gallon cans of alcohol to sell. If they thought the Mounties were around they tied a rope to a buoy with a bag of salt and then dropped the alcohol outside the harbour. When the salt dissolved the alcohol popped up and the Mounties had gone.

"That summer I relieved in Burgeo and Port aux Basques hospitals for six weeks. I was the Public Health Nurse in Ramea and did house calls in the morning, held clinic in the afternoon and then did house calls again. There were just over 1,000 people in Ramea, but Grey River and Duck Cove down the coast were also in my district. I'd hire a boat in Ramea to go there.

"There were no telephones except in Ramea. Mrs. Penney had a phone in the fish plant office so most messages got through on ship-to-shore. I took a patient to Burgeo and got a message saying someone was sick in Ramea. When I got back and checked things out, I realized there wasn't a medical emergency and the doctor didn't need to come because the doctor didn't go unless it was necessary. I got on the ship-to-shore and asked someone listening to their radio to tell the doctor to go to the fish plant to get a message. There was one car in Burgeo and no cars in Ramea, and we walked everywhere, so he had quite a walk to get to the plant.

"I always did what I was taught in training. If I did a home delivery of a primapara [first child], I visited twice a day for three days, every day to the ninth day and alternate days to the 14th day. With multi-births, I visited until the ninth day. My husband said that people in the districts got more attention after delivery than women in hospital where they were discharged after five days.

"I delivered twins in Ramea. I couldn't get a second fetal heart because of hydramnios [excessive amniotic fluid] so I had the doctor check. He wanted her to go to Burgeo for x-rays but people didn't have the money to pay $2.00 a night for board and lodging. In 1955 that was a lot of money! The woman said, 'What difference did it make if it was one or two? They would come when they were ready.' I had to decide the best thing to do because if we took her to Burgeo, she could deliver on the way and we would have to carry her on the stretcher over the dirt road. The logical thing to do was keep her comfortable in bed and wait. It was early and several women came to support the woman in labour. They put on a pot of soup and played cards in the kitchen. The first child delivered around 3:00 a.m. I thought, 'This will soon be over.' But when I palpated her there was another one, and three-and-a-half hours between deliveries! Their weights were 8 ¾ and 9 ¼ pounds. One was named after me and one after the Maloneys' daughter. They were Doreen and Maureen. We had a lot more patience then. I remember a woman from Grey River whose husband was the only one who ever came back after the delivery and asked how his wife was. The others went to have a drink with their buddies. I never forgot him.

"In Ramea we had clinics on Sunday, because what else was there to do only go for a walk? To paint the chairs in the clinic's waiting room I had to scrape off the gum from underneath. So I put a notice on the wall. 'The chairs are to sit on, not to park your gum. Please refrain from doing so.' For the next couple of weeks I'd hear them reading the sign, but it worked. The stove in the kitchen was a pot burner where the oil came into the wicks but I had never seen an oil stove. One day my housekeeper, who was 15 and had left school because this was the best paying job in Ramea, said, 'Miss Janes, I couldn't make your lunch because the stove went out.' I got someone to come and he was eight hours fixing it! The next time I got an oil blockage, I rigged up a piece of rubber tubing, with a glass connection and catheter. I sucked the oil up into the glass connection then blew it down again. It worked! I saved time and expense for the department. I also learned to deal with the plumbing for convenience. A lot of people in Ramea still carried their own water. I was lucky because I had a government house with a well, electricity, and 25-watt bulbs in the ceiling. The fish plant supplied our electricity. Half an hour before they switched off the power at night, they gave three blinks of the lights so you either went to bed or put on the oil lamps.

"The night watchman, who was diabetic, had a little wooden shack on the wharf with a pot-belly stove. His wife was concerned because he never saw a nurse or doctor and his teeth were in desperate state. I said, 'Don't worry. I'll deal with it.' One night I went with the dental instruments and said, 'Sam, you're going to have your teeth out. Do you want any anesthetic?' 'No,' he said. When I'd pull a tooth he'd spit into the pot-belly stove and I threw the tooth in. I did this until the offending teeth were pulled. Many young people then had no teeth because there were no dentists. Young girls got married with no teeth. Those whose teeth were all right went to the mainland because their fathers worked on the draggers.

"Something that amazed me was photographing the dead in their caskets. We had a boy, about seven, who drowned in Ramea, and I saw a photograph of him in his casket on the wall in the kitchen. There was no funeral home then and I was called to re-plug a body I had laid out. As I went into the house someone was coming out with a camera! I laid out a man in Placentia. He was big and lay on the floor. His sons were amazed at how I maneuvered and rolled him to get him dressed. This is an art that has long since gone.

"I went to a house on the furthest point in Ramea because somebody was choking. You can imagine I got there as fast as I could! An elderly lady had taken TUMS and started choking. I couldn't take her to the nursing station to suction so I took my stethoscope apart and used the tubing ... it was common sense. When you haven't got things, you make do!

"I got a telegram from the doctor in Burgeo requesting me to go to an emergency in Grey River. I hired the boat *Castaway* in Ramea because the hospital boat *John Kent* was out of commission. Captain Cutler said we'd leave at daylight because the cross currents were dangerous at night. While there, I visited almost every house in Grey River and brought two people to the hospital. I got drugs from the hospital in Burgeo and the doctor escorted me back to the boat. There was only one light on the wharf and as I stepped from the *John Kent* to the *Castaway*, the boats parted and down I went. I couldn't swim. I imagined my family getting news: 'Lost off the Coast of Newfoundland.' Luckily the doctor grabbed my arm and hauled me aboard. Everyone laughed! The doctor got dry clothes from the nurse: a plaid shirt and slacks, too big for me, and a camel dressing gown. I ran a high fever. The next day a 'dragger' was sent from Ramea to get a body. As I boarded the ship, the welfare officer shouted to the captain, 'Chain her on or she might go over again!' Sometime later the movie *Captain Courageous* was shown in Ramea, and Spencer Tracy sang a song to a boy who had fallen overboard from a luxury liner called 'Don't cry little fish.' One day on my rounds, two boys saw me and started to sing this song!

"I was in Ramea for one and a half [years] of a two-year contract. I said I would stay a third year if I could go to a hospital. As it happened, Dr. LeGrow had requested that I return in charge of the Channel hospital. Jean Lewis thought if I agreed there'd be no more complaints because he liked UK nurses. I planned to travel after that but we got a new assistant medical officer, which is why I'm still here.

"Although Channel was classified as a four-nurse hospital there was often only two. The nurse-in-charge gave anesthetics and I taught the new doctor, my future husband, open-mouth anesthetics for tonsillectomies because he'd never done that. I pulled teeth because the previous assistant refused to do it and would send for me. I taught the other nurse how to pull teeth and unfortunately she pulled one for me.

"Dr. Crookshank did relief in cottage hospitals, and being a good Scotsman, George went up on the Channel hospital roof to play the bagpipes. Patients would ask, 'Miss Janes, would you ask the doctor to play the pipes?' He also got a home-brew recipe from someone in Channel and made it in the bathtub. It took the surface off. You don't hear these stories now!

"Nurses lived in the cottage hospitals, and there was a doctor's apartment which had two bedrooms, a sitting room and bathroom. One part of the nurses' section was for nursing aides and maids. The other half had four rooms allocated for nurses. When my husband came he set up a semi-kitchen because he wasn't used to the Newfoundland diet. And you had to get used to it! I was introduced to salt fish and scrunchions in Ramea. I thought salt fish was like our smoked fish. I remember one dinner of chicken with vegetables boiled in salt meat! Another thing that fascinated me was cutting a portion out of the bologna. But I didn't realize it was cut to lie flat until I cooked a piece.

"Channel hospital had 34 beds with a male and female ward and a couple of private rooms. We had a visit from Dr. Leonard Miller, who was in charge of cottage hospitals. We were at the desk getting report when one of the nurses said, 'He's here. What do we do?' I said, 'We'll pretend he isn't here and carry on as usual.' He wasn't a very big man but you couldn't pretend he wasn't there! We did a round of every patient. I insisted on that because often something springs to mind that you mightn't think of in report. Then we all went for breakfast in the dining room. Evidently it impressed Dr. Miller because he wrote, congratulating me on the running of the hospital, and he wasn't in a habit of doing that!

"My husband came in May of 1957 and I was leaving in October. I went back to England because of the isolation in the outports, and if I was to marry it was for life. We were engaged while I was in England, but Newfoundland needed doctors so I came back. We didn't tell anyone we were engaged, and John was in Norris Point and I was posted to Old Perlican.

"When I arrived the new hospital was half built. The nurses' rooms had doors but no knobs. I was in bed one morning when the door opened and one of the workmen came into my bedroom and put on his overalls! At one stage there was a wooden ladder to the next floor and at the top of the ladder was an unhooked toilet sitting in the middle of nowhere. It was crazy! During construction Dr. Wilkinson continued to do surgery, and the evening clinics were crazy. He carried his own drugs and if you sold his, the money went into one of the elastoplast cans on the shelf. Money for the Department of Health drugs went into another, and money for teeth went into another. Western Bay didn't have a doctor so the people from there paid $3.00 and that was put into another can. They took the receipt to the hospital board in Western Bay and the money was refunded. One day someone from the Department of Health found the books were crazy, and selling drugs was stopped.

"We were married in April and a doctor's position in Placentia became vacant. We were there for 10 years. I never officially nursed there but I worked with the Red Cross. I started Well Baby Clinics, and at Christmas I babysat in the hospital while the nurse on duty went to midnight mass or when the Mission Fathers came so the nurse could go to the mission. I kept in touch that way. There was a doctor from England who brought his own boat and went around to the communities. He charged more for his drugs than the Department of Health doctor, so people preferred his because they thought the more expensive drugs worked better. He showed movies in the little settlements and told John, 'I always have a Western because you're guaranteed another clinic the next day after the young ones beat one another up doing what they saw in the movies.' He was a real character!"

❉

Doreen (nee Janes) Ross was born in London, England. She completed a course in fever nursing (RFN) in London in 1949. She graduated as a SRN from Royal Sussex County Hospital in Brighton, Sussex, in 1952 and completed her SCM at the Simpson Memorial Maternity Pavilion in Edinburgh, Scotland, in 1954. She immigrated to work with the Department of Health and after a period in Stephenville Crossing cottage hospital was posted as Public Health Nurse in Ramea.

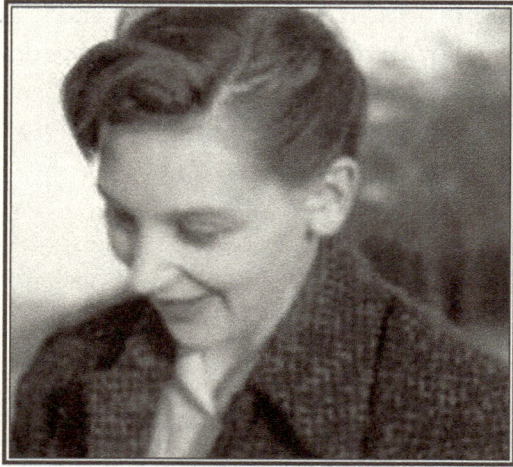

MURIEL (BUCKLE) MICHAEL

❋

1956

*"There were lots of English nurses who came to Corner Brook
and probably 50 to 60 percent of them stayed. Many who came said that
they'd go back to England to retire, but none of them actually did."*

"The Korean War was on, but I was rejected by the army because my father died of tuberculosis. They were afraid to send me to a tropical country so I came to Newfoundland instead. I waited another year and worked in a chest hospital doing TB testing before coming to Newfoundland. I was 25 when I arrived with two friends.

"The hospital in Corner Brook was much more modern than anywhere I worked in England, but it was small, so in a month we knew every nurse there .... I worked on the male floor, which had medicine and surgery. There were four rooms with two beds each and a ward with six bays and four beds in each and a big hall down the middle. We got patients from the Northern Peninsula but not quite as far as St. Anthony because they went to St. Anthony hospital. There was no road, so patients came on the coastal boat, usually by themselves. The coastal boats stopped when the ice came, and while I was there four or five patients got stuck in Corner Brook for the winter and their families spent the winter without them. The hospital was a memorial to the war veterans and was built through subscriptions from the general public and probably Bowaters.

"I worked until I got married, less than two years. I married a friend of an English doctor who worked at the hospital. My contract was for two years and if I worked more than a year, my fare was covered, so I was okay. The two nurses I came with completed their contracts, then one went to Saskatchewan and the other back to England.

"I had four children, which kept me busy for quite a few years. Then I developed nerve deafness that gradually got worse. When my youngest daughter started school I wanted to go back to work, but hearing aides weren't very good then. The ENT doctor thought it would be dangerous for me to work because I might not hear doctors' orders over the phone properly, or things like that. I worked as a volunteer at the hospital for about 30 years, because it didn't matter how deaf I was.

"I've lived here twice as long as I lived in England. I only went back to England once, but my mother came here every two or three years. There were lots of English nurses who came to Corner Brook and probably 50 to 60 percent of them stayed. Many who came said they'd go back to England to retire, but none actually did because by then your children are grown and married and you have grandchildren here. In my case, almost everybody I knew in England is gone.

"I enjoyed being a nurse and regretted that I could never go back full-time. My nursing experience in Newfoundland was not nearly as good as nurses who went to the cottage hospitals. One nurse, who trained at the same hospital as me, went to Harbour Breton, which was completely cut off then, and another one was near Wesleyville. She told me that if a patient was transferred to Gander they fought to get on the helicopter to get out of Wesleyville. Their experience was much broader than mine. Many of us regretted not knowing about the cottage hospital system because we would have enjoyed it, not forever, but for a limited time. That would have been a wonderful experience."

�֎

Muriel (nee Buckle) Michael was born in Raweliffe, England, and graduated in 1950 as a SRN from the General Hospital in Sheffield, England. She completed her SCM in Middlesex Hospital, London, England, in 1951. She finished a course in Tuberculosis Nursing in London in 1952 prior to immigrating in 1956 to work at the Corner Brook Western Memorial Hospital.

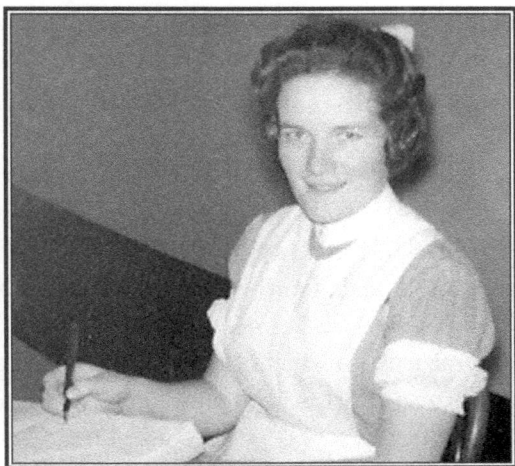

MARY (SHORT) ROUSSEAU

❋

1964

*"It was pitch black and I was stuck in the back seat
between two big, burly men. I had no idea where I was going.
I could be going to the ends of the earth!"*

"We wrote to places all over the world to see what was offered. I wrote to Corner Brook and forgot about it. I was interested in Corner Brook because of the skiing. They wrote me about nine months later and asked if I was still interested in coming to Canada. I also applied for a job in Gibraltar and was in the process of getting my English registration. But Corner Brook offered a ten-month tour of duty, so I thought, 'While I'm waiting, I'll come to Canada, do the 10 months, and by then I'll have my registration and I'll go to Gibraltar.' I made my travel arrangements myself. It was the first time I'd flown. I stayed overnight in Glasgow and had never stayed in a hotel by myself before. I was in this big cavernous room, which was scary. I flew into Gander and from Gander on to Stephenville.

"My mother said before I left, 'I don't want you going away, you must come home to live.' That was a period when there was a lot of out-migration from Ireland and my mother knew people whose family left and only came home infrequently or didn't come home again. I don't think she visualized I would be home every other year.

"From the literature I got, I assumed a limousine service was going to meet me. I sat in the airport waiting, and a taxi driver came up to me and said, 'Ma'am, where are you going?' He knew I was a foreigner because I had no boots and there was snow on the ground. My husband always jokes about the fact that I arrived in Gander in a little pair of gold suede shoes and there was about a foot of snow on the ground. I said, 'I'm going to Corner Brook but I thought a limousine would meet me.' He said, 'No, I think this is the only limousine service.' It was pitch black and I was stuck in the back seat between two big, burly men. I had no idea where I was going. I could be going to the ends of the earth! The only thing I knew about Newfoundland was where it was on the map of the world. Eventually we got to Corner Brook and he dropped me off at the nurses' residence on West Street. Somebody put me in a room and I'm thinking, 'Oh my God, what have I done?' The next morning I woke up and it was like a village from a storybook because of the snow on the hills in the background. It was really pretty, my impression of an American village.

"I went to visit the Director of Nurses, who said, 'We have to get you registered here in Newfoundland.' And I said, 'I'm already registered. Here are my forms.' I had decided that if I didn't get registered before I left Ireland, I wasn't coming. So when I got registered, I didn't have a choice. Getting nurses registered after they arrived apparently was the norm, and people had to work as graduate nurses until then. But I knew registration was important to get full salary, so I did it before I left.

"They said they'd fly me out and fly me home and that was all I understood. When I got here I realized that the local nurses were getting two days off a week, but I only got one day off a week because my contract was for 10 months. Apparently if you stayed a year you got two days off a week, but I didn't think that was specified in the literature I got. I was only here a month or two when I said, 'I'll stay for the year, but I want two days off a week.'

"I arrived at the hospital the next morning, was interviewed and taken to pediatrics. People in administration were quite business-like but friendly. They sent me to work on pediatrics, which wasn't my area, but I thought I'd try it because I'd done pediatric orthopedics and thought it would be all right. I didn't get a real orientation to pediatrics. I got some but it was very skimpy and on the job. I was on peds three weeks when they decided they needed somebody in the OR, and I had OR experience. I didn't find the OR friendly and it had to do with the head nurse. She was gruff and business-like to everyone, not just those from a different country. The system here was based on the British system and there wasn't a whole lot of difference. There wasn't a lot new in the OR because the policies and procedures were very alike. Within a short period of time I got to know everybody. There were some Irish doctors who were friendly and I got used to working there. The working life really wasn't an issue. The case room was just outside the OR. We did all the cesarean sections and I did not think the practice of obstetrics was very good because it didn't seem that the nurses in the case room had very much control. But every hospital has its little nuances and its own culture.

"But I found the nurses were, 'Oh God, we have a new nurse that we have to teach the ropes to!' There was a kind of jadedness towards new nurses who weren't trained in the Canadian way. They weren't unfriendly, but coming to a new country you need to be pampered in the beginning to make you feel at home. It was lonely in the beginning because I knew nobody and had come here alone.

"But I was lucky because I met the Rousseaus three weeks after I got here and they were a very friendly family. Also, there was another Irish nurse here who was friendly, and there were families who invited us out. I found the people you met in the street were very nonchalant. 'Oh, you're from away.' That was it. The people in the community were more open for our presence than the nurses. The people I got to know were marvelous. The Rousseau family had a different culture, but was very outgoing, friendly, and really nice and had a similar value system to mine.

"If I said I was from Ireland, people here would say, 'We're all Irish, but where do you come from?' What they meant 'What part of Newfoundland are you from?' I got that reaction a lot of times. People say Newfoundland is close to Ireland and friendly. But to me it was obvious we came from different cultures. I came from a very Catholic background, and even though my School of Nursing wasn't Catholic, the staff there were mostly Catholic. They were like me because we all came from the same culture and background, which was a rigidly Irish background. I had to get used to different cultures, different perceptions and different ways of living. I was very naïve and not very worldly, so I found somebody living with somebody a bit on the strange side. I was a little sanctimonious! I'm sure it happened at home but I had never been exposed to it. Another thing was somebody coming in beaten up with bruises, and everyone would go quiet and not talk about it. You'd ask what happened to the person and somebody said, 'Her husband probably beat her up.' Again I'm not saying it didn't happen at home, I'm sure it did, but I wasn't exposed to it. There was an Irish doctor on staff and one day he was in the lounge telling dirty stories. When I came in he said, 'We'd better shut up! Here's Holy Mary!'

"When I came, Corner Brook was like a village. It wasn't even as big as a town in Ireland, but I thought it was a beautiful village, a very pretty place with mountains. And of course I was fascinated with the snow and loved the idea that we have snow for so long. I really wanted to learn how to ski. That was one of my main reasons in coming to Canada. I had this image of being able to ski and doing outdoor winter things. I just loved it, and also it was really a great way of getting to know people, and where I lived was quite nice, as were the girls in the residence. But I was into reading *The Irish Times* or *The London Times* and current magazines. Here you'd get something that was a month old! I couldn't believe you couldn't get a magazine that was up-to-date! People thought I was a bit pretentious. There was a little newspaper here, *The Western Star* or whatever it was called at the time, and I'd think, 'Don't you have any world news?' because I was really into news and current affairs. Even as a young person I was interested in that sort of thing.

"I lived in residence for a year and a half until I got married, which was quite nice. There were lots of nurses from away, Canadian, English, and Scottish girls who were very nice. We are still friends. There was one Canadian nurse who was really funny. We were foreigners in her place, but she was sweet, really grumpy but a good egg.

"I always wanted to travel and really loved being a nurse. I did nursing in the very beginning because it would enable me to travel and it was a method of getting a job anywhere. I planned to travel several years before I settled, but then I got married to a Newfoundlander. But I did think long and hard about the fact that I would be living here for the rest of my life.

"I go back to Ireland almost every second year so I've been able to maintain that contact."

�֎

Mary (nee Shortt) Rousseau was born in County Meath, Ireland. She graduated as a SRN in 1962 from the Royal City of Dublin Hospital in Dublin and completed her SCM (Part 1 and 2) at the Rotunda Hospital, Dublin, in 1963. She immigrated to work in the hospital in Corner Brook in 1964.

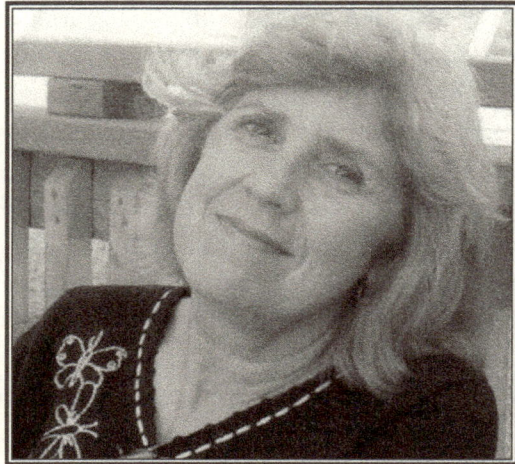

KATHLEEN (COLLINS) HEALEY

❋

1974

"I couldn't get registered. I was given a temporary registration because I had only done six weeks of psychiatry and I needed three months."

"My husband found out about Newfoundland from a medical journal looking for residents at the new medical school. In those days it was good to spread your wings. It took us 23 hours to fly from Heathrow to St. John's. It was a milk run, stopping in every Atlantic province— Montreal, Prince Edward Island, everywhere. We had two small children, 11 weeks old and three years. Thank goodness for breast-feeding! In those days, when coming on an international flight to St. John's, you got off the plane in the middle of the tarmac. We were up to our knees in snow. I didn't have boots because I had no idea what to expect. Then we went to Marystown, where my husband was supposed to start work after a few days of acclimatization. A snowstorm happened there and we were at the Mortier Hotel for three days. My husband went to the house where we were to live. He came home for lunch and said, 'We have to go back to St. John's because they can't find the stop cap to turn on the water in the house. There's too much snow!' So we went back to St. John's.

"Then 'between the jigs and the reels,' as they say, we went to Harbour Breton, which was four hours from Grand Falls. The journey was amazing. There was nothing but dead blackened trees and snow on an unpaved road. In England, at least you see houses. Harbour Breton is on a bay and when we arrived it was like a fairyland. It was about 4:00 p.m. and the tops of the mountains were pink and the houses were different colours and the lights were coming on. It really was a beautiful spot! But the next weekend was a totally different story with a terrible snowstorm. They lost a snow plow! We had no electricity in the house, and four of us snuggled in bed because it was the warmest place. We lived on peanut butter sandwiches and orange juice. It was a very interesting bonding time.

"After a couple of months there, I went to work because the nurses at the hospital were working 16 to 24 hours a day. I worked night duty and my husband and I did alternate nights for three months. On my first night, a lady was having her sixth baby and the doctor was doing a high forceps delivery. The patient kept saying, 'Am I making a fuss?' I'd never seen anything like it. She was a wonderful person and I doubt she had any more. The stoicism of these people was just amazing. I really enjoyed working there.

"We were there five months. The doctor was considered like God, which amazed us. We never saw such a hierarchy before. We met the Anglican minister, the judge, the fish plant owner, the social worker, the other doctor and the customs officer—all the professionals. They were the only people we got to know well and we made some good friends. We were introduced to other people, but it was difficult to get to know them. I always tried to engage them in conversation and would have loved to have a cup of tea with them, but it just wasn't going to happen, which was a shame.

"We learned a lot about the social life in Newfoundland. The interaction of the churches was interesting, on one side of the bay was Catholic and the other side was Protestant. But if the Anglican minister ran out of palm crosses he borrowed from the Catholic. That was wonderful. We also learned a lot about the seasons, how the fog, the cod and capelin follow each other and then the berries come. It was a cyclical thing. Harbour Breton was a wonderful experience and we left just before the berries came.

"We went into St. John's to find an apartment. It was 70 degrees and we were in shorts. Two days later on our way back, we stayed overnight in Clarenville. The next morning there was six inches of snow on the road, which was disheartening. But by the time we got to Harbour Breton it was gone. That was the first time I experienced snow in June.

"I couldn't get registered. I was given a temporary registration because I had only done six weeks of psychiatry and needed three months. I had worked at a famous neurosurgical and psychiatric hospital, but I did six weeks in neurosurgery. I sat the exam and I failed, so I couldn't get registered. I had three children and didn't study. Also my husband was working alternate nights and alternate weekends. I found St. John's very lonely. We had one or two good friends, but I found it very difficult.

"We moved to St. John's in July '74, and we needed money so my husband could go home to finish his residency. His mother came for three months to care for the children while I worked full-time night duty. I worked at St. Clare's and found it very different from nursing in England. We had taped reports for a start! And the nurses didn't do as much of the care as I was used to doing. I was on the gynecology ward and the first few nights a lady said, 'No one did my bandages today.' She'd had varicose vein surgery. I'd been trained to first do a round of all the patients to make sure they were comfortable and settled for the night. Then I'd do the dressings that hadn't been done during the day, but I could never understand why they hadn't been done. Also I wasn't trained to do IVs, because at home we had medical students, so I had to learn how to do them and I got my certificate. But the 12-hour shifts were hard. We had so much more responsibility and didn't push paper like they seem to do now. After I did three months on the temporary licence, I worked as a call-in nurse and specialled patients when they needed someone. I did that for about a year at St. Clare's and I loved it!

"After three months, Chris' mom decided it was just too much. She didn't drive and had the children until I came home. She would keep me up talking until about ten o'clock and I'd have to go pick up our oldest daughter from pre-kindergarten at 12:00 noon. I'd go to bed for a couple of hours in the afternoon, then I'd have to get up, cook supper and go to work. I was younger then but it was really hard.

"We'd been here a year, so we all went to England when my husband went to do his exams. There were daffodils up there when we came back here in early February to snow half way up the door. My husband came back here to finish his Canadian fellowship, but by the time we were ready to go back to England in '77, it was very difficult to get back because things had changed so much. Then my husband got a job in Corner Brook. The people were amazing, absolutely wonderful, and after six weeks we decided to stay. We were made so welcome and it seemed such a beautiful place with so much opportunity for the children. It was Easter and there was still snow on the ground, but that didn't put us off because we loved the snow. We skied in Austria and wanted to teach the children to ski. Also we loved to canoe and camp and hike, so this was a perfect place for us.

"I couldn't work. The Director of Nursing here wasn't very co-operative. I had my teaching certificate but she said, 'If you want to register you have to go away for a year. I won't let you work here.' So I did the MCP billing for my husband. Then we had our fourth child and my husband set up his own practice and I worked on and off in the office. I didn't do much when the children were small, but once they finished high school I worked more. I did all letters, billing and accounts, and kept things up to date. When our last child went to university I did an afternoon antenatal clinic and did blood pressures and counselling for the moms. I work more often now and do the swabs for pregnant women and that kind of thing. It has been wonderful. I really miss nursing and the patients. I've wanted to be a nurse since I was five years old. I could never imagine a time when I didn't.

"Our families were in England. We used to go back as often as we could, but with four children it was very expensive and there were other things that we wanted to do. I did a degree in English and we travelled with the children. I don't regret coming here. I love Newfoundland. My husband retires in another couple of years and when he retires I'll retire too."

❊

Kathleen (nee Collins) Healey was born in Peterborough, England. She graduated in 1965 as a SRN from King's College Hospital School of Nursing, London. She completed Midwifery, Part 1 in 1967, Dulwich Hospital, and a Clinical Nurse Teacher Certificate in 1970 from Royal College of Nursing, London. She immigrated in 1974 to Harbour Breton with her husband, a physician.

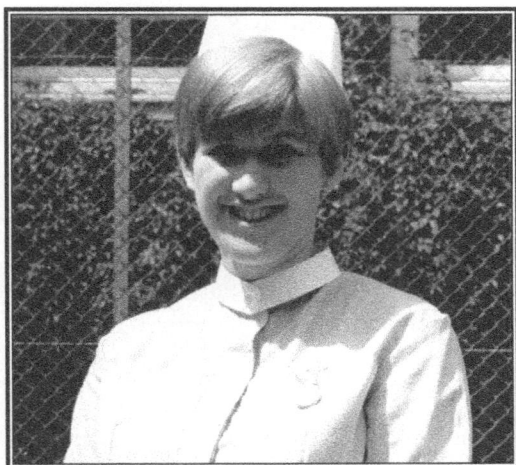

KATIE (BLIGHT) WATTON

❋

1967

"I found the informal nature of working here good because there wasn't this strict adherence to rules whether they made sense or not. There was more focus on the patient and patient care, which was refreshing, and I enjoyed it."

"My girlfriend and I became ward sisters at a fairly young age. I was 26. It was a nice job but probably not going anywhere soon because we were so young. One day she saw something in the *Nursing Times* that said they wanted nurses for three months in this place called Corner Brook, Newfoundland. I thought, 'If I don't do anything now, I never will.' I knew Newfoundland was around the Grand Banks, and Dad said it was the cornerstone of the empire and that was what I knew about Newfoundland. We weren't interviewed. It was a purely paper application. We sent proof of our RN and SCM to Human Resources at the hospital and that's all we did. They arranged everything else.

"I came into Gander with a group of 27 nurses and we got on a proper CN bus. We stopped at the Baie Verte junction to get a cup of tea in the Irving Station. When we got out, all you could see was 360 degrees of trees, no houses, nothing! It was Father's Day. We also stopped in Windsor where the signs said, 'Make Pappy happy' and 'Make dad glad.' We thought this was hilarious and roared with laughter. In Corner Brook we came down Brookfield Avenue and saw tiny individual houses made of tin. I'd never seen Alcan siding and thought, 'Isn't this bizarre?'

"We were brought over in response to a nursing shortage. They housed some of us in Maple House, which is where I was, and some in residence. They paid our way here and if we stayed the three months they paid our fare home. Also the pay was better than in England so that was incentive in itself. To be honest, I didn't know the geography of Canada that well, and I thought I would be near other attractions and I'd be able to travel more than I could in fact. We had very little idea of what we were coming to.

"They did a very good three-day orientation for us. They took us to the new hospital that was built but not functioning. They explained procedures and the Director of Nursing spoke with us. We were asked which area we wanted to work in. I was open and went to surgery, which suited me fine. They utilized the skills of everyone who specified an area. I was pleased with our reception from the nurses. There were differences in nursing and we had to get used to each other. They were very receptive but you had to be a little careful. It was a case of 'When in Rome do as the Romans do.' Some things shocked me and other things were done quite well; you had to be tactful.

"I was horrified at the way drugs were dispensed, and when I talked to the others, we all were. It was a disaster waiting to happen! In the hospitals at home, drugs were dispensed directly from a doctor's order and taken to the bedside. They were never transcribed. Here the orders were transcribed by somebody, put on funny little cards with the patient's name, which then sat in little Dixie cups that were taken around on a tray. I was stunned and couldn't believe they were allowed to get away with this. That was the biggest difference I found. There were different names for drugs, but we were up to par with that within a couple of weeks.

"The team work was very good. I was used to a hospital with student nurses but here there were only graduate nurses on staff and I enjoyed it. Also the head nurse was less aloof than I was used to in Britain. She was one among many but part of the team, and I found that good.

"It was strange that everything was referred for the doctor's opinion and I'd think, 'Good gracious, what business is it of his? This is a nursing matter.' The nurses here had very little autonomy in their own field. Doctors would write orders like 'Care of the feet' and I'd think, 'Of course you're going to do that. The patient's a diabetic! Why would he write that?' because that was nursing, not medicine. Also the hospitals I'd worked at had residents and interns and the ward sisters knew a lot more than they did and guided them. Here we only had consultants.

"The dialect was difficult to understand, especially on the telephone when speaking to visitors or patients from outports like Burgeo, who had really strong accents. I would have to say after the third attempt, 'I'm terribly sorry! I'll get somebody.' My ear is good now and I can speak to anyone.

"When I was first doing surgical interviews, I'd had to ask people how many children they had. My first patient, who was a little sliver of a lady, said, 'I had 18.' I thought, 'She's pulling my leg!' But I got used to that after a while because some had up to 22 children. I'd never experienced that in my life. My great-grandmother had 12 and that was the most I'd ever heard of. I was bowled over by the huge families.

"The patients were charming and very nice. I suppose people were nice to us because we were different.

"Initially I wasn't keen on Corner Brook. I found the fact that everybody knew everybody really disturbing. I'd always lived in an anonymous society, but here your movements were tracked and I found it bizarre, but I don't even notice it now—I probably do it too. I missed the theatre and things I did in London. I missed shopping because there was no shopping here then. Also there was nowhere else to go different. Once you're in Corner Brook, you're in Corner Brook unless you go to St. John's or Stephenville, whereas in London I could go to New York or to different places within England.

"Many nurses who came bought white uniforms because that's what the nurses here wore, but one of the group wouldn't adapt and wore her navy belt with the white uniform. Knowing I was only going to be here three months, and, in fact, there were 27 of us, helped me adapt. It affected how we integrated and the way we coped. We were a novelty item in town for three months.

"I returned to England after my contract ended and I did some shift work with a nursing agency. I wore a pantsuit and one night this austere Sister said, 'Would you please not wear your pajamas to work?' I found the informal nature of working here good because there wasn't this strict adherence to rules whether they made sense or not. There was more focus on the patient and patient care, which was refreshing, and I enjoyed it.

"I never had a problem with the nurses but some of the doctors were a little different. One had illegible writing and I refused to transcribe one of his orders. I said, 'I can't read your writing and have no intention of taking off orders if I don't know what they are.' He really got snippy with me because they weren't used to that, but my head nurse backed me up. I was pleased with that.

"In the middle of the three months I met my husband and soon realized this was different. He had to go back to law school in New

Brunswick and my contract ended in September. I went back to England and in November of the next year I came back, got married, and started working at the hospital. I didn't give leaving home much thought, I was so sure I wanted to get married that everything else paled. It impinged on me greatly when I realized what I'd done. I had a couple of rough years wondering if I'd settle in, but then you have children and it becomes your life. My parents were good about my coming here, although maybe a little shocked I didn't get married in England. They didn't meet my husband until the night before we got married. We got married in St. John's because my husband's family was there.

"But it was totally different when I came back to stay, although my welcome was just as enthusiastic. I never had a problem with working. I have roots here now. It's my home and I wouldn't go back to England to live. I've made good friendships and the people here are the friendliest in the world. I like being here and I like my lifestyle. My parents both died and I have no reason to go back, but I do to visit my girlfriends. I'm invested in Canada and became a Canadian citizen."

❋

Kathleen (Katie) (nee Blight) Watton was born in London, England. She graduated as a SRN in 1970 from Middlesex Hospital School of Nursing in London. She completed the SCM, Part 1 in Farnborough, Kent, and Part 2 on the Isle of Wight. She immigrated to work at the Corner Brook hospital in 1975.

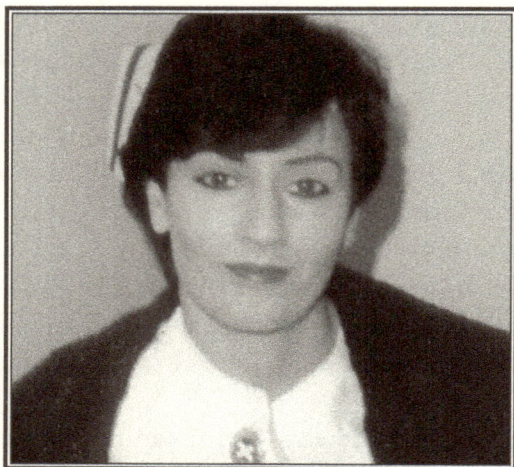

RUTH (BURNS) LAMB

❈

1983

*"I flew into Gander and had a connecting flight to Stephenville.
The airport there was about the size of my dad's shed!
I thought, 'This is a big mistake!' If I had a credit card then,
I'd have been on the next plane."*

"I was waiting to get in a neurology course so I applied to different places. Corner Brook was the first one I heard from. I came home one day and my mother said, 'You've got a telegram (which you did in those days) and it's from this place Newfoundland to offer you a job in Corner Brook. I don't know where that is.' And I didn't know where it was either!

"I came because there was a big nursing shortage here. There were about 40 British nurses recruited at the same time. I didn't know anybody but I was young and it was something different. They gave us a place to stay and paid our airfare and said, 'If you like it we'll extend your visa.' I got the visa from Glasgow and the hospital here looked after the registration and everything else. When I told my parents I was coming, they were devastated. But I was 22 and only coming for a year, but my mother knew the difference. She's never forgiven me.

"I flew into Gander and had a connecting flight to Stephenville. The airport there was about the size of my dad's shed! I thought, 'This is a big mistake!' If I had a credit card then, I'd have been on the next plane. I told somebody at the airport I was going to work in Corner Brook and asked, 'How do I get there?' They told me there was no bus and I ended up paying for a taxi from Stephenville to Corner Brook. You just assume this is how it is. I arrived on Sunday. I went to the front entrance of the hospital and said, 'I'm here to work and I don't know where to go.' They told me to go to the residence and ring the bell and they'd show me. I had no contact with anybody from the hospital until the following day. If someone had met me and said, 'Welcome to Canada! I'll take you to the residence,' I'd have felt more welcome, but there was nobody. I phoned my father and said, 'This is a big mistake!' I would have gone home, but I shared a room with an x-ray technician from St. John's who had family in Corner Brook. She took me under her wing and said, 'Come, meet my family and we'll have something to eat.' That helped but the hospital could have done a lot more.

"It was very lonely and I didn't understand what people were saying because I found their speech very thick at first. Also, some of the terminology was different; the money was different with the tax to be added. It was little things like that. Also it was difficult finding the shops.

"Corner Brook was a very closed community and very old-fashioned. People would say, 'You're from Scotland. I suppose it's very much like here.' They really didn't understand just how different it was to come from another country. But they were very accepting, very nice and very open once you got to know them. The nurses were great and I did feel welcomed.

"The big things for me were the cultural differences and loneliness. There was no group of British people. If there had been someone to take you around the community to show you where you go for groceries, the drug store, or a list of taxis, it would have eased things tremendously.

"I was only here a couple of days before I had to go to work. I went to work in medicine, but two weeks after I got here they said, 'We're really under a crunch. Would you help us for a couple of months in psychiatry?' I had three weeks of psychiatric experience as a student, so this wasn't my preferred area. One of my first patients was a lady who thought she was a cherry tree. I really felt inadequately prepared to deal with this situation, but that's the way it was. You were put where you were needed.

"I came from a big teaching hospital and things were very regimented. Everybody had a uniform and you knew who was a registered nurse, a sister, doctor or an x-ray technician. When I came here I had no idea who anybody was because the doctors didn't wear lab coats, and in psychiatry everyone wore street clothes. The whole approach to nursing was very laid back compared to Britain. On one of my first shifts, at nine o'clock at night, somebody asked for a lunch. I'm thinking lunch is in the middle of the day and couldn't grasp that they meant a snack. Then they had Carnation milk in their tea! It was very different.

"I had difficulty with drugs because of the different names. Somebody would say Tylenol, and I never heard of it and people didn't understand why I didn't know it. Also if a doctor wanted to examine a patient, he'd ask for a flashlight where I knew it as a torch, and if I said torch, nobody knew what I meant. Also I had never taken telephone orders before.

"The biggest difference was that GPs ran the hospital. It seems normal to people here because they've always done it that way, but I never understood how a GP could come in, look after patients, then go home at night, and only one GP was on for the whole area. It was a totally different system from what I was used to in a teaching hospital. It took a while to get used to.

"I came for a year but after 10 months enough nurses had graduated from nursing schools, and basically they told us we could get lost and pay our own air fare back. It left a bad feeling. I had met my husband but wasn't overly involved at that time, so I went home to work in a nursing agency in Edinburgh. But my husband and I had started a long-distance telephone relationship and I ended up coming back. I got married, had three children, and stayed home with them. About eight years ago I did the re-entry program and came back to nursing. I was never registered here because when I came, I worked on an interim licence.

"It is very isolated here, and although I was married, I thought, 'I'll just jump on a plane,' but with children it's not that simple. Until I started to make friends in the community it was very difficult. After a while, I met some war brides and got involved through the children and with neighbours who had children. At first my parents were able to make the journey but they're older and my father's not well. I go home often but find it hard to go home and have to leave. I'd go back to Scotland in a heartbeat. I have no family ties here because my husband isn't from here, and once my boys get older they'll have their own families."

❋

Ruth Lamb was born in Dunfries, Scotland. She graduated from Southwest Scotland College of Nursing and Midwifery in 1981 with a GRN. She immigrated in 1983 to work at the hospital in Corner Brook.

Chapter Three

ST. JOHN'S

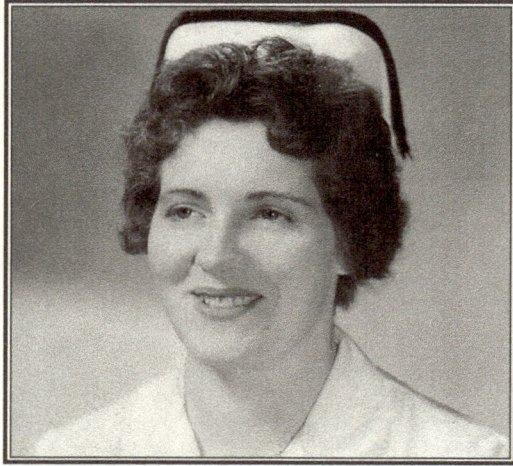

MAY (KERNS) McCLOY

❋

1957

"We came in February on the SS Newfoundland *and ours was the worst journey across in 50 years. The boat had to cut through the ice; it was treacherous!"*

"A nurse in Dublin told me about her two years in Newfoundland. Later I saw an ad saying they were recruiting nurses at a local hotel. A bunch of us decided go. The interviewer was a man from Dublin and very strict. They checked our references and asked what we'd like to do and where we'd like to go. I had no problem getting a nursing licence and my references were good. My mother thought it was good to travel and it was only for year.

"Five of us came and were very happy taking a voyage on a ship. We were told we'd sit with the captain for breakfast and that the food was good. We came in February 1957 on the SS *Newfoundland* and ours was the worst journey across in 50 years. The boat had to cut through the ice; it was treacherous! I was so seasick; I said, 'That's it for me. I won't be going back by boat.' We spent the time saying our prayers because we thought we were going to die and that's the truth! For my first meal I was asked to have breakfast with the captain. I thought, 'That's great!' It was kippers. That was the first and last time I ate kippers.

"A nurse met us at the dock. I asked to go to the sanatorium because I had a vocation to care for people with TB but was told I'd be going to the General Hospital. We were taken to the hospital cafeteria. I wasn't accustomed to that because at home staff nurses were served in the dining room, a big treat. They had fish and brewis. I'll never forget it! After such a terrible journey! Then we were taken to the residence and introduced around. It was my first time sharing a room. The girl was from Ulster and when I knocked to introduce myself, she was reading her Bible. She was Protestant. I had worked with people of other faiths, but she was frightened to death because I was the first Catholic she'd met. But we became good friends. When I went for the interview my mother said, 'Ask if you can practice your religion.' What a question coming to Newfoundland! But I asked the right nurse, Mary Feehan, about church. She said, 'Your church is St. Joseph's down the road. I'll get your church envelopes.' I'd never heard of church envelopes and thought Newfoundland was way ahead of Ireland.

"I worked on Alexander children's ward which was enjoyable. There wasn't much orientation. I met the head nurse, assistant head nurse and the pediatric nursing instructor. After a couple of hours on my first day, I said to another nurse, 'Has anyone put on the kettle? Shall I make the tea and toast?' She said, 'We usually go to the cafeteria but that is a good idea. We'll get everything done quicker.' That is what I did in the

UK. When the doctors finished rounds, the student had the tea ready, and we talked things over while we had tea. So we kept doing that on Alexander.

"Alexander babies were young. They called it the prem unit. On nights and evenings we had 40 babies and a nursing assistant with me. Doctors and interns often helped us feed the babies, which was nice. If a doctor called at 11:00 p.m. and said, 'I have a child to bring in,' I had to find a bed even if the cots were full. You never left the floor on evenings. It was madness with the IVs and everything else. We did a lot of shifts, like 11 evenings or 11 nights and then got a day and a half off.

"I got a call one night from an American lady asking if any of the nurses would like to come to dinner, meet her family, and do a little babysitting for them. She went off to the American base and came back with a couple of fellows to party. One was a lawyer and I became friendly with him. None of us drank or smoked, but we loved dancing. He invited me to the Officers' Club for dinner, and when I went there was a lobster sitting in front of me. I had never seen lobster, never mind knowing how to eat it. I said, 'You'll have to fix it for me.' He liked that because I didn't put on any show. He was a great talker and used big words. When I'd get back to residence after going out, the girls would say, 'What's the new word you learned tonight?' One night he said 'in the vernacular' and I never forgot that! I was thrilled when I found Lawlor's butcher shop because I could get real bacon, liver and other meats I liked.

"We lived in residence at the General until they moved us to make room for the students. That was a sore spot because the Americans were here and it was difficult to find a place. I moved in with a group of nurses. I said to the landlord that I hoped the apartment wouldn't be too hot, which was a big mistake, because we nearly froze to death. Also it was haunted! I woke up to a nun sitting on my bed! Later the local people told us they also thought it was haunted.

"I spent a lot of time walking to places like the gut. We went fishing with the fishermen and cooked [the fish] in residence. Also, local church groups invited us to afternoon tea and we'd have fashion shows where nurses modelled clothes. I joined the militia for 12 or 13 years and got the rank of captain. A group of us went to Camp Gagetown, and after that we went to Montreal for a holiday. We had a good time at the regimental dinners.

"There wasn't a lot of difference in nursing here and at home. There were different drugs but we could look them up in a book or ask people to help us. I didn't have any problems. I worked on Alex until my contract ended and would have returned to Ireland but I met my husband. I went to the wedding of one of the nurses who married a fellow who worked with my husband. A friend of his gave us a ride and that was the beginning. My husband is from Winnipeg and was working with the Marconi Company when I met him.

"The American woman took us shopping at the base. We met different people through them and had a lot of fun. She made my wedding dress because we didn't have a lot of money then. My salary here was about $50.00 a week. I got more in Ireland because I worked in a TB hospital. She did a great job. It was satin, which I bought for $10.00. My one bridesmaid was one of the UK nurses and I still write to her. I married in April '58. Her husband gave me away and someone replaced my mother. None of my family came. My mother wouldn't fly then, but she came later and stayed for six months and was godmother to my second youngest. The wedding was in the morning at the Basilica. Everyone at the General was there, a couple of hundred people. We had a do at Bidgood's.

"Towards the end of our contract we were interviewed by the supervisor. She said, 'I reviewed your papers and we need someone to teach microbiology and communicable diseases,' and I had done that. I could have gotten any job, there were so many choices, but I took the one at the Fever. I had gotten married in the meantime and was pregnant. The nurses gave me a baby shower. They wanted me to go to the Grace for the baby and I did. I worked during my pregnancy and the baby was born with no ill effects, although we did have polio there. After that, I had to stay home then because my husband travelled. It was sad giving it up, but the nurses visited me.

"After four years I went back doing casual on nights or evenings. You could work whatever hours you wanted. You'd never be without hours. Then somebody from the Janeway said, 'Why don't you do a few hours with us?' I remember one nurse coming to the house when I was in bed, asking me to go to Intensive Care. That's how short they were. The nurses never left the babies. They never went on break. Someone would get you a cup of tea, but that was the way it was.

"I went back to work full-time in 1975, teaching nursing assistants at the college because there was a shortage. That was a great place to work. Then I worked at St. Patrick's Mercy Home and got my degree (BEd) while I was there. Then I went to work at Exxon House and there were talks of closing it. I got transferred into the Waterford. Let's just say I found that challenging! Then I got a call about a permanent position at Hoyles Home and I went there.

"I haven't been home for six years because my husband can't travel. Then my son died suddenly and that takes its toll."

❁

Mary (May) (nee Kearns) McCloy was born in County Mayo, Ireland. She graduated in 1951 as a SRN from Milend Hospital School of Nursing in London. She completed Midwifery as a SCM, Part 1 at Milend Hospital in 1952 and Part 2 at Hammersmith School of Nursing in 1953. She completed an Operating Room course and a Registered Tuberculosis Nurses Certificate before immigrating to work at the St. John's General Hospital in 1957.

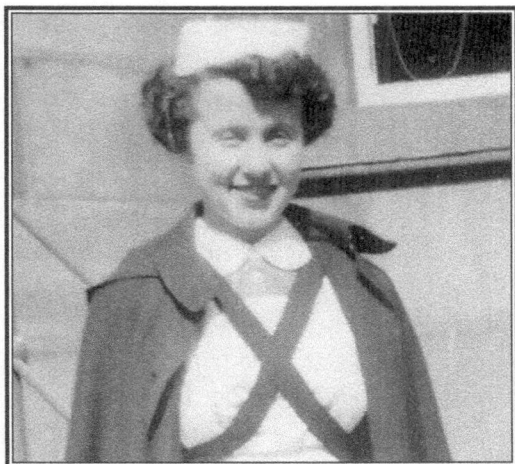

ANNE (HARKIN) BAIRD

❀

1961

"Mr. Shaw put everything in motion with the Newfoundland government;
he arranged everything from this side …. I didn't have to do anything."

"The Newfoundland government was always recruiting staff from over-seas and their agent, Mr. Shaw, was in Liverpool and travelled to Ireland, Scotland, and England recruiting. He gave talks and we were young and wanted an adventure. A lot of the nurses went to Boston and a lot came here. I hadn't the vaguest idea where Newfoundland was. I spoke Gaelic so had learned about it in school, but we called it *Thalamh an Eisc*, the land of the fish.

"I was working in Glasgow when my friend and I talked to Mr. Shaw. Then she upped and married my cousin. Everyone said, 'Now you won't go.' But I thought, 'I'm going.' When you're young, you don't see obstacles.

"Mr. Shaw put everything in motion with the Newfoundland government; he arranged everything from this side. I had to contact the register for nurses in Scotland, get the medical clearance and get inoculated. The shipping company arranged the travel. They were excellent. I was told, 'This is where you go, and what you do.' I didn't have to do anything. I had no problems getting licensed here because I had the general nursing and midwifery.

"Mr. Shaw gave me the name and address of an Irish nurse here and suggested I write and she would bring me up to date on what I needed to know. We corresponded about six months, so I knew some-body when I came. She said that a lot of the people from Ireland went on to Boston. She was in contact with them and they really liked it and maybe I should consider Boston. It was a subtle hint!

"I travelled alone. I didn't know a soul in North America except the nurse I'd been writing to. My mother was dead and my father had remarried, so I was free and looking for adventure. I signed a one-year contract because I didn't plan to stay. They paid my way out for one year and would pay my travel back if I'd stayed for two years. It was a chance to travel first class on the SS *Nova Scotia*. I was given a choice of Corner Brook or St. John's. I figured the General was a larger hospital so I opted for that, but I wasn't prepared at all for what it was like here.

"I wasn't met by anyone. It was July and the fog was down to the waterline! All you could see was the Battery. Two people I got to know on the ship were British and lived here. They said, 'That's St. John's up on the hill where those houses are.' I said, 'It can't be! I'm coming to work in a hospital!' And they said, 'Behind those houses is the hospital.' I thought, 'My God, where am I?' I went through customs in an old shed on the waterfront. I stood there with my suitcases strung about me when the two people came along and I said,' I don't know what I'm supposed to do.' They dropped me off at the hospital and somebody showed me where the nurses' residence was. They said to go there and somebody would contact me later.

"I remember standing in the room and looking at the American Base. I never felt so lost in my life. I kept saying, 'My God! What have I done?' I was alone for hours before somebody came and took me to the nursing office. They didn't tell me much, except I had to work the next day. I was still weaving from being on a ship for five days! I had to purchase a nursing cap and white shoes, which they suggested I get downtown. I was issued a white uniform that was way too big for me. I had to take an oath of allegiance to the Queen because I would be a civil servant, but I said, 'Sorry, I didn't come all this way to do that!' They said, 'You have to, to be employed in Canada.' I said, 'I worked in Britain and didn't have to take an oath of allegiance to the Queen and certainly won't do it here.' My father would have a conniption; he was jailed by the Queen's father. I said, 'The ship is still in the harbour and I can go back on it.' I didn't mind going back at that point. There was a hustle and somebody said, 'We have the same problem with some Irish doctors. They swore allegiance to the government of Canada.' I said, 'No problem, I can do that.'

"They suggested I go downtown to get white shoes, but I never found downtown. I walked down Forest Road and was hungry, so I went into a store and asked for a package of crisps. They didn't know what I was talking about. I thought I was in a foreign land because they didn't speak the same English. I was supposed to ask for potato chips. I wandered down Duckworth Street and a little boy had raw stuff in a box with flies all over it. I asked what it was and he said 'flippers.' I've never eaten flippers since. I never did find a shoe shop so I came back.

"I met an Irish nurse on the floor who lent me a pair of white shoes. They were too big but I managed for a week. Nursing veils weren't worn here so we got a generic cap and put a black plastic ribbon on it so people knew we were registered nurses. The next morning I wore the white shoes, which were duty shoes, and tied the uniform around me like a sack. When I found Water Street, I bought uniforms that fit!

"Someone brought me to Three South where I was to work. The head nurse said, 'I'm so glad to see you. I haven't had a holiday in two years!' I said, 'You're not going now?' and she said, 'No,'—but she did go in two weeks. She left me with a nurse doing a refresher course who hadn't worked for 10 years. I was frightened to death because I was responsible and didn't know what I was doing. When I came there were 27 RNs at the General Hospital, including faculty, and third-year students were doing a lot of the work. You didn't get an orientation to things like policies and procedures. So after the head nurse left, I called nursing office asking, 'What do you do in this situation? What's the ruling on this?' But they didn't seem to know either and would say, 'You decide what to do and let us know.' I think they were far removed so they didn't know either. There was no one to fall back on.

"Three South had the only private rooms in the hospital, and with no ICU, sick patients went there. We had coronaries patients in oxygen tents. One patient had chest pain and the doctor wanted morphine. I couldn't find any in the cupboard and said, 'We don't have any.' The Ward Clerk said we did. She took me to the utility room and unwrapped a package which had a metal container. 'Put the pill in there, squirt some sterile water on it, and mash it up.' I'd never seen morphine pills given intramuscularly! I'm trying to mash the pill and the doctor is screaming for the morphine! The ward clerks kept me sane because they were able to tell me everything I needed to know. Everything was different, especially drugs, like demerol, I was used to meperidine. I would ask for a pipette and that was a medicine dropper. It's a different language, different terminology, different way of doing things, and different routine.

"The older nurses watched me but didn't get too friendly. I think they felt we thought ourselves better than them. We did things differently and did say, 'Why are you doing it like that?' Nurses had no autonomy. There had to be a doctor's order for everything and we weren't used to that. If a lady's feet were cold, you had to have a doctor's order to give a hot-water bottle, because I did that and got in trouble! It was in case it was inadequately done and the patient got burned. I thought, 'Train the nurses to fill the hot-water bottles properly.' But that never changed. If someone had a headache I needed an order for 222s and also for laxatives. In Scotland, we didn't. We recorded when patients would need a laxative. Here I was always on the phone tracking down a doctor because we couldn't take a verbal order. I got in trouble; we all did. We were too independent, but that's how we were trained. It was aggravating.

"Also I wasn't a big fan of doing bed baths every day. In the UK we had a team. We did surgical rounds and showed students and nursing assistants how to do dressing. Then we let them do it on their own and checked later. Here, you were isolated. You went off with your list of three or four patients and that's all you did. If you were concerned, you had to ask somebody to have a look and tell you what they thought. We'd only see each other at coffee break. We had one supervisor who made a fuss about dust bunnies under the beds! That was what her round entailed, not the patients.

"For the first six months I truly hated it. I had the calendar and I marked every day. I did meet the girl I had been writing to and she had an apartment with three others and one was leaving. She asked if I wanted to move in with them. I lived in residence to that point, and most evenings the conversation was about the best way to polish wax plants. The sheen was a big issue. We also talked about the best solution to get white shoes gleaming. I was 20!

"Once I moved in with the other girls I had someone to talk to and had a social life. First when I came, nobody tried to involve me in things. Newfoundland has a reputation for friendliness, but it's at a distance, removed a level. Everybody speaks to you, but they've been with the same people since school. They went into nursing with them, are in card clubs together, and they don't invite you into that. You were always on the outside.

"Mary Feehan grabbed us as soon as possible because we were Irish and Catholic. She hauled us to the Catholic Nurses Guild's meeting every month and showed us St. Joseph's Church and what time mass was.

"I won't forget my first Christmas here. It was horrendous! There were three of us on a 30-bed, acute care floor with a full patient load. Christmas Eve we admitted two coronaries who were in oxygen tents, a fractured hip, and two young fellows who crashed their car, and one had to have a craniotomy. He came from surgery with a tracheostomy which had to be suctioned every 15 minutes. The medication had to be given, the dressings and treatments had to be done. It was a nightmare. I was worried about the patient with the tracheostomy because I wasn't getting around to suctioning him. But the patients survived despite us. We had an old fellow with a fracture who had to go to the OR. I had prioritized and decided he was the least of my worries, but his doctor wanted him immediately and came to see if he was ready for the OR, I said, 'No! I haven't got his skin prepped; I haven't got anything you need.' But he wouldn't wait for me to get him ready. He went into the patient's room, pulled the bed, Balkan frame and all, and ran down the corridor. There were mirrors over the desk so we could see what was happening in the corridors. The doctor caught the mirror in the Balkan frame, and it fell and broke into thousands of pieces, raining down on the old fellow's head and he was screaming. Everybody ran out of the rooms to see what was going on. The doctor didn't pause! He just pulled him through the double doors of the OR, bed, mirror and everything. This went on in the middle of patients we were trying to keep quiet, especially the coronary patients.

"I got a taxi home at four-thirty in the morning because I couldn't leave the nurse who came on at midnight. I came back at four the next day and the other evening nurse had called in sick. The supervisor said, 'Nowhere in the city is there a nurse to be found.' I didn't have time to be homesick! I didn't go to mass. It was just weird.

"Mary Feehan in the nursing office would say, 'You girls would love to see the outports!' We didn't know what an outport was! She had us escort patients home who couldn't make the trip alone. That was very interesting because you'd go on the coastal boats, mostly around the south coast. She didn't warn me that there were no nurses or doctors anywhere and when people heard a nurse was in port they'd arrive. But I didn't have anything with me! I was supposed to diagnose, treat wounds or dog bites, all kinds of stuff. I could only advise them about what to find locally because I didn't come prepared. It was surreal!

"One time in Rencontre we picked up a patient in labour who was supposed to go to Harbour Breton. I had to leave the lady I was escorting and go down with this woman, who was pushing and was almost ready to pop the baby out. I said to the captain, 'We better go straight to Harbour Breton,' because I didn't think they should stop at the ports along the way. When we got there the only transport was a gravel truck because there were no roads. The hospital was on a hill so we lowered her onto the gravel in the truck. I had to kneel in gravel in case the baby arrived before we got up the hill.

"I had a patient in Terrenceville and there was a lot of fog. We had to stay overnight and were in the big waiting room in a boarding house where everybody waited for the boat. It was packed! I put the patient on a chesterfield in the corner and looked after her there. She had to use the bedpan so I got some women to stand with their backs to her while she used it. Everybody was gawking and trying to see what I was doing. I had to ask them to look some other way. The bathroom was upstairs and I had to march past them to empty the bedpan. Also the poor lady was throwing up! We couldn't get into the small island she was from so we lowered her into a dory from the side of the ship. It was scary but fascinating, and I loved doing it but it was a crazy night.

"I was definitely going to go home but met someone and got married. I debated whether I should go back anyway, but by then I had friends and had gotten into the swing of things and it wasn't so confusing. My family didn't come over for the wedding and my friend's husband gave me away. We had formed our own little community and could talk about things we knew. I could call them and ask, 'What do you generally do with this?' even with nursing, and we'd decide what to do. It was our support and there wasn't a lot of support otherwise.

"After I married we moved to Placentia and I volunteered with well-baby clinics twice a week. We'd weigh the babies and give mothers advice on feeding. We handed out cod liver oil and orange juice. I remember one gorgeous baby from Fox Harbour and I asked the mother, 'What do you feed him? He looks so healthy! She said, 'Slops!' When she left, I asked the nurse, 'What's slops?' It was bread soaked in tea.

"We returned to St. John's in '67 and I worked at St. Clare's in pediatrics, then moved to the case room. I worked there until I had another baby in '69, because you had to give up your job then. I went to work at the Sanatorium because I lived in the west end and I liked working in the Sanatorium when I was in Scotland. I worked there until it closed in '73. I liked working there; it was a happy place for all the misery. There were three generations of families! Once Rifampin came on the market, patients were sent home with their pills and the place closed almost overnight. The patients left were transferred to St. Clare's and the staff went with them. I was Evening Supervisor at the San, so I moved to that position at St. Clare's and was there until I retired. It wasn't retirement really, it was redundancy.

"Looking back I should have gone to a small community or up in Labrador because it was more the kind of nursing I did at home. You had more autonomy and independence and could use your initiative more.

"I go back to Ireland every year. I stay with my cousin. She's my connection over there. My three children live in Canada."

❄

Anne (nee Harkin) Baird was born in Donegal, Ireland. She graduated from Chalmers Hospital School of Nursing, Edinburgh, Scotland, in 1958 as a Registered Graduate Nurse (RGN) and completed her SCM at the Royal Glasgow Maternity Hospital in 1960. She immigrated in 1961 to work at the St. John's General Hospital.

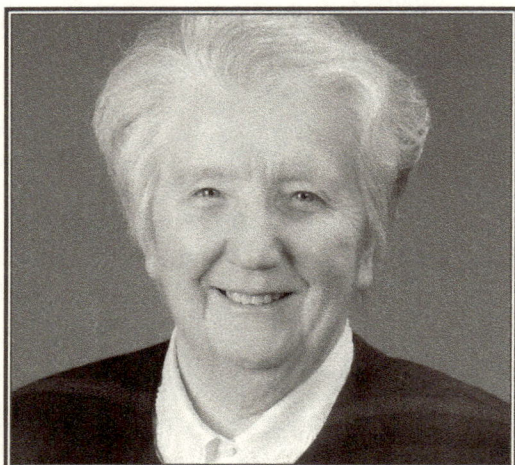

KAY (KIELTY) MATTHEWS

✳

1967

*"Maternity practice was very different here. What I
found hardest was that here you had to get the doctor."*

"I was born in Ireland, but my family moved to England when I was
seven. After I graduated from midwifery, I worked in Oxfordshire where
I married my husband and he dragged me to Newfoundland. He was
recruited to the university. He came home one day and said, 'We're going
to Newfoundland.' And I said, 'Where's that?' I had two babies at that
time. After I got here I had two Newfoundlanders.

"I had trained in the Lamaze Method for helping women during
labour and childbirth. After I had been here a few years I had women
and their husbands at my house to do the course so they could manage

labour better. The method wasn't known here at the time and women got opposition from Labour and Delivery nurses. I thought, 'If you can't beat them, join them.' I did a refresher course at the Grace and discovered they expected a shortage of staff that summer. I applied for the case room and got employed there.

"Maternity practice was very different here. What I found hardest was that here, you have to get the doctor. I felt particular pressure to make sure the doctor was there or they'd think I was trying to be a midwife. I found I did more internal examinations. Also, I had to learn to scrub for caesarian sections, which I hadn't done in community midwifery in England. For the first three, I would say to the obstetrician doing the caesarian, 'This is my first one, doctor,' so that they'd be patient. Once baby and mother left the case room here you didn't see them again, so if it was somebody I sat with, I tried to pop down to the floor to see how they were doing. Here, there were a lot more inductions and interventions, which wasn't common in England. But there was great camaraderie in the case room. I enjoyed my colleagues and loved nights when we sat together at a quiet time, and we'd talk about our experiences and what it was like training as nurses. It was hard to believe the Atlantic was between us because nurses are the same across the world. We tend to stick together and most are very collegial and like working with people. That part was really enjoyable. I was accepted by the nurses, although there was suspicion at first because I was a midwife. They thought I'd come with some queer ideas. I clearly came from away, but they forgave me! I consider it important to get on well with my coworkers, so I tried not to create any awkward situations. A sense of humour helps a lot. The health care system here and in England is very different but the principles are the same. After three months at the Grace, I felt comfortable.

"I had no problem with the accent. But one thing that amused me was when family phoned in and said, 'Is she better yet?' Meaning, 'Has she had the baby yet?' That was a bit different.

"I worked in the case room at first and then got the position of maternal/child health coordinator to develop the parent teaching program. I set up prenatal classes, post-partum classes for in-patients and then established the breastfeeding outreach clinic. I resigned because my husband was going on sabbatical to England, and when I came back I decided to complete the nursing degree. It took me 15 years to get my BN but I got my master's a lot more quickly.

"After finishing the BN I worked at Memorial and at the same time I also ran the prenatal program at St. Clare's and the Grace. My husband died in '84 so I started the master's program because I had to earn some money. Then I got employed full-time at MUN and stayed until I retired in 2002.

"I go back to England quite frequently. I've been working in Africa since '92 and Indonesia since '85. In Africa I was the nursing and midwifery consultant for Africa Care and we ran safe motherhood projects in Nigeria and Ghana. In Indonesia we ran a project in nursing education and women's health from '87 until 2006. Now I'm in Nunavut training Inuit women as maternity care workers.

"Newfoundland is my home. I still call Ireland and England home, but certainly Newfoundland has been a major part of my life. All my kids consider themselves Newfoundlanders and we all are Canadian citizens.

"I had a wonderful nursing career in Newfoundland because I got to do everything. I was in a clinical practice, research, teaching, and on the Council of the ARNNL. Nursing in Newfoundland is in excellent hands. I can't speak highly enough of it."

❋

Kathleen (Kay) (nee Kielty) Matthews was born in County Tyrone, Northern Ireland. She graduated in 1960 as a SRN from St. Anthony's Hospital in North Cheam, Surrey, England. She completed midwifery (SCM) in 1963 at General Lying-In Hospital and the Churchill Hospital, Oxford, England. She immigrated to St. John's in 1967 with her husband who was recruited to teach at Memorial University.

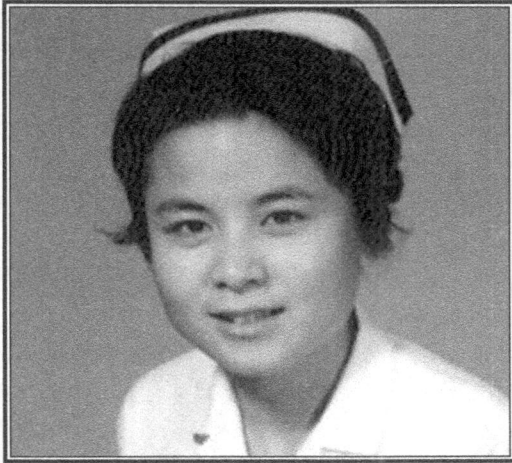

LAN (NGUYEN) GIEN

❉

1968

"You have to make what you're doing more interesting for yourself.
Nobody is going to make it interesting for you."

"I did my nursing education in the USA. In the '50s and '60s, the US government wanted to create influence in Vietnam so they gave scholarships to people completing high school, to go to the States. You had to pass English to get a scholarship and I learned it in high school. My father didn't want me to go. He wanted me to stay home and get married. If I didn't get a scholarship, I couldn't study anymore. At home, then, if a girl got an education it was difficult to get married. I took the exam and passed. A lot of people didn't want to go to the States because it was so far away and strange. People wanted to go to France because it had been with Vietnam for a long time. All the good students went there. I don't know how my father agreed but in the end I went.

"It was quite difficult. There was another person with me so we hung onto each other. At that time there weren't many people from Vietnam and if you said you're from Vietnam, they'd say, 'Where? Vitamin?' There were about 100 of us on scholarships. We were so lonely that a Catholic priest in Chicago took pity on us and created a book of the students' addresses and sent it to everyone. It was like a Bible! We were so happy. Everyone became instant friends.

"I left the States because I wasn't a permanent resident. My family was in Paris and I went there to work. In Paris there was a huge population of Vietnamese. When I met any I'd say, 'Hi! How are you?' They said, 'Are you nuts?' They didn't need the kind of friendship that I was hungry for. I worked there for over a year in an acute care surgical area but the difficulty was I had to speak French.

"I got married and my husband was recruited to work at MUN. I was a new bride with no children. I had nothing to do and was looking for work. I got a job at the General Hospital School of Nursing, my first job in Canada. I told Miss Story I had just graduated and didn't want to teach, but I had no choice, that was the only position available. I asked about the pay and she said $4,000 a year. I said, 'When I worked as a student in the States I got more than that!' She said, 'We are a poor province.' But I wanted to work anyway so I didn't care what I got. But we saved money. We rented a basement apartment for about $100 a month. A cup of soup cost 10 cents. We still had a car. I saw apartments on Elizabeth Avenue and went and told them I wanted to rent one. They were public housing for people on welfare! But I didn't know the difference. We lived in a basement apartment for two or three years before I found out that there were apartments in Pleasantville. I called and they said, 'You have to put your name on a long list.' But I knew someone who was moving out so I said, 'Can I move in?' and I got it. Life was simple then.

"I taught the med-surg course. I had to teach classroom and clinical. I did a lot of clinical. Planning and trying to prepare the lessons was a big challenge because it was all new and I had to teach in English. I didn't realize how much time it took to prepare a lesson. I worked day and night because I did a class every day. There were 120 students and we used a microphone because the classroom was so big. I didn't have a problem with students speaking. They laughed at my accent and I didn't know why then. They paid more attention because of my accent. I told them they had to write clearly, otherwise I wouldn't understand. They couldn't skip words or drop words and expect me to understand. That helped their writing. I wasn't much older than the students, and later we all had children about the same age. My daughter came home from school one day and said, 'My friend said you taught her mother and that you were so funny.' Maybe my accent kept their attention, but I think they were friendly.

"Miss Nicholle was the director then and every day she stood in the door and if students had their skirts above the knee, she told them to take the hem down. Or she said, 'You're late!' She was very strict. But the students respected her and she was warm-hearted. We only had one car and she often gave me a ride to MUN.

"Nursing here was different from Paris but I was surprised that nursing here was not that different from what I had learned in the States. I had trouble with some patients who were difficult to understand, but in general I had no problem. I worked at the General Hospital for five years. Teaching nursing was busy and if I had a day off, I was happy. They were nice at the General Hospital and we made friends so I didn't feel lonely.

"When my husband went on sabbatical I did my master's. Also I had to be in Canada five years to become a citizen and get a passport so I could travel freely. I came to Memorial University, but teaching at the university wasn't very different. The semester system is different and we could plan family time better. Also we didn't have as many students and every summer we worked two months in the medical-surgical area, so those that taught med-surg worked almost year round. There were only six people on faculty.

"We were the first Vietnamese in Newfoundland. Our family grew up here and we stayed. I have no regrets coming to Newfoundland. I still work at the university and it's been a good career. I don't regret being in nursing. I tell my children nothing is perfect. You have to make what you're doing more interesting for yourself. Nobody is going to make it interesting for you.

"I guess the story is, if you want more nurses to come here, then you have to recruit their husbands."

❋

Lan (nee Nguyen) Gien was born in Vietnam. She graduated from Loretta Heights College in Denver, Colorado, with a Bachelor of Science in Nursing in 1964. She emigrated from Paris, France, in 1966 with her husband, who was recruited to teach at Memorial University.

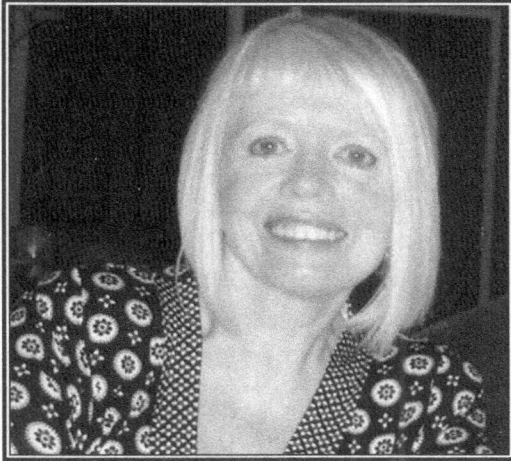

GWYNNETH JONES

❋

1974

*"When we arrived in St. John's there were 37 of us
that went to the General. We all came on the same flight but
we didn't know each other until we arrived."*

"They were advertising for nurses to come to Newfoundland for the summer to work, and my friends and I thought, 'That's a great way to see Canada!' And the pay was a lot better than what we were getting in Britain. We thought we'd save enough to go to Australia.

"We travelled from London to Edinburgh for the interview. The interviewer offered me a job in ICU because I had an ICU course. I didn't want to work there, but I felt I wouldn't get the job if I said, 'No,

I'd rather do medical nursing.' I agreed to go in ICU. The paperwork was all done for us. We got less money because we didn't have full registration. We had to have a medical. I did not have psychiatry, which was an issue with licensing of overseas nurses, but I got my licence because the ARNNL brought in a by-law that nurses could get licensed provided they had psychiatry or obstetrics. I had OBS. English girls didn't necessarily do psychiatry in their nursing program, but Scottish girls had both. We came on interim certificates but once we decided to extend our contracts we were able to get licensed.

"We came because we were young and wanted to do something different, to see a different aspect of nursing, and the pay in Britain was about $2,000 a year and here the pay was $7,000. That seemed a big difference. And if we didn't like it, it was only four months.

"I came alone and sat with an Irish nurse I did my midwifery with. We met at the airport in Manchester. When we arrived in St. John's there were 37 of us that went to the General. We came on the same flight but we didn't know each other until we arrived. We stayed on the seventh floor at Southcott Hall; we paid $21.00 a month—very little. We had to provide our own meals.

"My first impression when I landed in St. John's was that it was quite cold. We all brought summer clothes because we heard it was hot in Canada. It snowed on June 7! And all the houses were wooden. We weren't used to wooden structures; our houses were bricks and stone, very different. But it was quaint and we liked it.

"The crowd that were over the year before us were partiers, and some nurses in ICU thought, 'This crowd is only over to party. They're not here to work.' They found out we were better. The younger nurses couldn't believe our average age was 25 and we weren't married; 37 single women!

"Our orientation wasn't very long, maybe two days and that was it. We arrived on a Sunday and started on Monday. The staff was good but the ICU was extremely busy. We were thrown in and didn't get any significant orientation to the area because we were there for four months, so they weren't investing a whole lot. I had an ICU course and the other girls had worked in an ICU, but everything was very different. The names of the drugs were different, the names of the procedures were different. We called a Levine tube a Royal's tube and demerol was pethidine to us. There was a fair bit of getting used to but not a lot of challenges. The general terminology used in the hospital and the charting were different. We had support within our own group and shared similar experiences versus people who came on their own.

"It was very different culturally. We used to watch *MASH* and compare it to what we were like. We had to buy white uniforms and shoes. At home we wore the hospital uniform provided. When we arrived, our uniforms were mid-calf length and other nurses had dresses above the knee and they were chewing gum! It was culturally totally different, more relaxed and very informal.

"One incident was very upsetting. We had a lady from one of the Iron Curtain countries and her husband was working at Come By Chance. She had a car accident and was in ICU a long time. When she died we found notes she'd written to her husband saying that we were really cruel to her. There weren't any names. We gave the notes to him, but it was very upsetting to realize how she had perceived us. When she wasn't intubated, her English was very poor.

"Shopping in St. John's was very poor then. Some of the people's fashions were a few years behind what we had. And food was very different. I lost 30 pounds in two and a half months because I just didn't like the food and in ICU we never got meal breaks and worked a lot of overtime. The staffing situation was terrible. I ate a lot of salads because the food tasted weird. We lived in Southcott Hall and didn't do a lot of cooking. Belbin's, a local grocery store, stocked British food and it only took us five minutes to walk there, so we'd fill up with stuff that we knew. It was nice and convenient. I managed to survive for four months and was in love by then.

"We used to rent a car to go places and we met people who took us to different things. Everything was new and we were all very anxious to see whatever we could. We'd go down to the Hotel Newfoundland and we'd go to the lounge there. I had one Canadian nursing friend from BC, but mostly we stuck together.

"I came at the beginning of June and I met my husband-to-be at the end of July. In two months my contract ran out so I went home with another girl and we packed up the rest of our stuff and came back. I decided to see how things went. I packed for winter. I was home only two or three weeks. Our work visa was for nine months when we came, so that was still in order.

"I didn't tell my parents I was going to get married but said I had met somebody. My mother was happy because it was closer than going to Australia. We got married in March. My friend's work visa was up and she got married because she couldn't get it renewed. If you got married you got an automatic landed immigrant status and you were okay.

"We moved to Gander in December '75 because my husband was going to open an office. I was very happy where I worked and liked St. John's, and I did not want to move to Gander. I had established a social life in St. John's. But my husband wanted to start a law practice by himself and in Gander there was only one law firm. I came under duress.

"He hadn't met my parents, so we went to England for three weeks and got back in January and I put my name down as casual. There were no permanent jobs so I worked casual on the medical floor. It was difficult because I'd never worked on a floor here. Then I got a permanent position in pediatrics and worked there for a few months until I got transferred to medicine. At that time we had 20 beds, two of them were private rooms with monitors. I came into work on my own time one day for the head nurse to show me around and show me the monitors. I went to work that night with only a nursing assistant. It was totally different. I didn't know what anything was and I was on my own!

"I found Gander very friendly. It was a nice hospital to work in. It was the same in the community. When we came here we figured we'd stay 10 years and move on, but it's been a good place to raise children. It's safe and there are lots of activities for them.

"I don't think the nursing care was as good in Newfoundland as what we were used to. There would be one nurse to four patients on ventilators in ICU because of the staff shortage. On weekends, people would phone in sick and they couldn't get coverage. It was pretty difficult. I found it better in Gander.

"I've enjoyed nursing over here. At home it's a lot more structured and disciplined but I don't think that's necessarily good for the patient or the staff. The hospitals have big wards with 24 people in them, and here, people are in four-bed wards at the most and the care is pretty good.

"My parents used to come every other year. We'd go home one year and they'd come the next. They really liked it here. We thought about going to Britain to live but went home on a visit and it was so busy and crowded, we changed our minds. My roots are here and I'm quite happy. I love the lifestyle but I don't like the weather. I've got muscular dystrophy and winter is a nightmare. When I retire I will go to England for a couple of months to get away from winter but I won't leave. My children are here and this is their home. Britain will still be my home, and I just love to go home, but ..."

❈

Gwynneth Jones was born in Lancashire, England. She graduated from Royal Infirmary in Manchester, England in 1970 as a SRN and completed midwifery (SCM) at Elsie Inglis Maternity hospital in Edinburgh, Scotland in 1973. She also completed a six month ICU course at the Royal Infirmary in 1971 and immigrated to work at the St. John's General Hospital in 1974.

SUE (HARDY) MICHALSKI

✳
1974

*"The first year I came we got a lot of snow and it seemed
to me that it was up to the wires. It was incredible! I took
pictures and printed them to send home. I called home saying,
'You've never seen anything like the snow here.'"*

"I came here with three friends. Before we came here we went for three months in Stavanger, Norway. It was interesting and we thought, 'This is neat, going places. Let's look across the ocean and see what's there.' We went to Canada House and inquired about nursing in Canada and the person that interviewed us said, 'It's funny you should come today because there is somebody here recruiting for Newfoundland.' We looked at each other and said, 'Where's that?' There was a lady there from St. Clare's. She said, 'Can you start as soon as possible?' and we said, 'When we get our immigration papers.' Apparently they expedited them and in three weeks we were all on our way here. That was 1974.

"We flew into Gander and came in on a yellow school bus. There were flights but they didn't coordinate with our flight so we came by bus. In England you are never far from a big place. On the drive in we didn't see any people, very few houses, and all we could see was fir trees and water. We looked at each other and said, 'Where have we come to?'

It was only when the bus rolled into St. John's and we saw civilization that we thought, 'Okay, this is our home.' That was an experience! We arrived here on June 30, a blistering hot day, and had no inkling of what weather in Newfoundland was like.

"They took us straight to St. Clare's and put us in the residence on high hospital beds which several of us fell out of! Opposite us was the chapel where the nuns came every morning, also when some of the girls were rolling back in from the night out. Later they moved us across the street to a house with doctors' offices in the bottom and we had the apartment at the top. We came to alleviate the shortage of nurses. They hired us for the summer months to give nurses holidays. We had a return ticket and a six-month contract.

"I'd come from a very busy cardiovascular intensive care unit where we had very sick patients. It was high tech and go, go, go, then I came to St. Clare's ICU and thought, 'This is a breeze.' It wasn't what I classed as an ICU. It was an extended surgical unit. Other nurses thought they were busy, whereas we said, 'Phew, we get a rest.' But it was fun and very different. Everybody was on a first-name basis and that was unheard of where we came from. It was much more liberal here and it was good. Even the doctors were on first-name terms and we thought, 'This is really different.'

"My manager was a lovely person and very good to us. We had a little mini-training session to orientate us and then we were put to work right away. My very first patient was a man from out around the bay and I did not understand him. We had different terminology for things; like a bedspread is a counterpane in England and a washcloth is a flannel. During his bed bath I made my first couple of mistakes and he got agitated. I kept saying, 'Can you say that again, sir?' He said, 'Why are you calling me, sir?' I still refer to men as sir. It's ingrained. So I asked him, 'Do you have a flannel, sir?' And he answered 'A what?' Then I said, 'I'm just going to get a counterpane for your bed.' And he said, 'What are you talking about?' In the end he got so frustrated, he said, 'Don't you speak the Queen's English?' We all thought that was a huge riot. It was so funny. People spoke fast and while we all spoke English, it was different.

"By the time the six months was up I had met my husband. That was a drawing card. I applied for an extension of my visa, but I had to go back to England because of the immigration rules. I went home at Christmas and came back in the middle of January. I came back to St. Clare's and continued working there. Then I moved to the General. One of the surgeons started the cardiovascular program in 1975 and they didn't have enough nurses trained in the field. He asked if we would transfer over and that's what I did in October 1975. The St. Clare's nurses said, 'You won't like it at the General.' But I did. I missed the girls at St. Clare's, but when I moved to the General ICU it was like family. It was a great place to work and wonderful people and I learned a lot. The head nurses were wonderful and the doctors in charge of the ICU were both English. There were lots of English and it was a little self-contained unit. It was more like the ICU nursing I was used to. I stayed there and moved up to the Health Sciences when the new hospital was built and have been there ever since. The only times I've taken off were for maternity leave. I've worked consistently for the same employer for more than 30 years.

"When you are doing any training in England they put you up in residence. Once you're a Registered Nurse, or if you do post-graduate training, they put you up in an upscale residence because you're not a student nurse. So it was normal to be put up in residence when we got here, but it was a big thing on behalf of St. Clare's Hospital. When I moved to the General they didn't put me up, I had to find my own accommodation. That was different.

"Also I wasn't used to the snow. We get snow in England, but not where I'm from in the southwest. The first year I came we got a lot of snow and it seemed to me that it was up to the wires. It was incredible! I took pictures and printed them to send home. I called home saying,

'You've never seen anything like the snow here.' I didn't have to shovel because I lived in an apartment but I walked a lot and I found it very cold. We didn't have any heavy clothes, coming from England, but everybody was good when I first came. I made lots of friends and people took me to their homes. Some said, 'Come and spend Christmas with us,' which was different from England because people are more reserved. No one would think of taking you under their wing and bringing you into their homes. We thought people were so friendly here.

"I like bedside nursing. I had opportunities to move but I like contact with people and I like what I do. The people I worked with have been great. I went from Intensive Care to Emergency in the early '80s, and I really loved it because you don't know what's coming into the doors next. Everything is different and your adrenaline gets up. I work in Post-Op Recovery now and I love that, too. I've worked in specialty units all the time. We have more autonomy in the specialized units.

"My family came to visit many times. My parents love it. My father goes for long walks and talks to everybody and thinks it's a great place. My brothers, sisters, even my grandmother, have been here. I really love it here. This is home. I go back to Britain now and I feel like a visitor."

❋

Susan (Sue) (nee Hardy) Michalski was born in Hampshire, England. She completed a two-year course in orthopedic nursing from the National Orthopedic Hospital in London in 1969, then graduated as a State Registered Nurse (SRN) in 1972 from St. George's Hospital, Hyde Park Corner, London. In 1973 she completed midwifery as a SCM in Scotland, followed by a six-month cardiovascular/thoracic diploma course before immigrating to work at St. Clare's Hospital in St. John's in 1974.

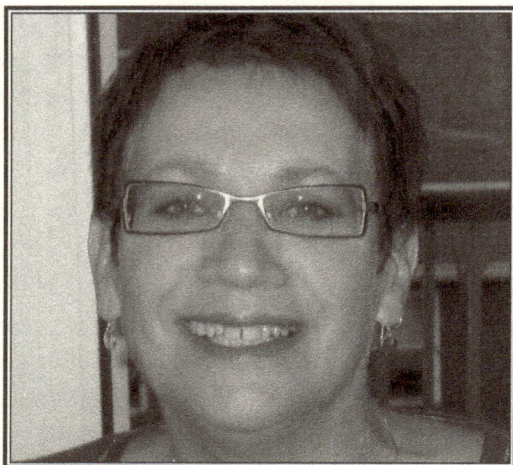

JO (BROWN) HENNEBURY

❋

1974

"We came on a school bus from Gander to St. John's. There was nothing really. It's like bare wilderness and I said to my friend, 'Oh my God, where have we come to?' I think everybody felt the same."

"My girlfriend and I got a couple of nursing journals and looked for jobs. She found the one for Newfoundland, but I said 'I've no idea where that is!' There was another one there for Portugal and we decided to apply to both. We went for interviews. I got a job for Portugal but my friend didn't, and we both got jobs in St. John's so we decided this is where we would come.

"On the way we realized there was a crowd of us. There were 30 girls from all over England and also several girls from Ireland. There was a bunch of girls at St. Clare's, a bunch at the Janeway, and more than 30 at the General around that time. We left on June 2 and arrived in Gander with snow on the ground. I was horrified! We came on a school bus from Gander to St. John's. There was nothing really. It was like bare wilderness and I said to my friend, 'Oh my God, where have we come to?' I think everybody felt the same.

"There was nothing really in St. John's in '74. The Avalon Mall was really tiny. There was no downtown scene. There was the Commodore Club and one or two other places. They took us right to the residence at Southcott Hall and we stayed together on the seventh floor. It was a relief. We signed a contract before we left and agreed to stay for four months, and they agreed to pay our airfare over and back. If we wanted to renew the contract afterwards, we could.

"There was no orientation. They went on your previous experience. I asked to go to emergency but there were no vacancies so they asked me if I would go to the operating room. I said, 'Yes' because I had some experience there but not a lot. But it was very hard, because there was no orientation, except on the job when you got there. And the surgeons were very stern, especially the urologist, and I was in urology. We circulated mostly but occasionally we had to scrub in. Nursing wasn't particularly different but I hadn't worked in the OR except in orthopedics. There were differences like the eight-hour shifts, which are all they did in the OR. We didn't do *call* because they wouldn't let us. We weren't qualified for Canada. We would have to write exams if we were going to stay. We were classed as graduate nurses, not registered nurses.

"After a couple of weeks we were out and about and the place to go for a night out was the Kellick Club at the old Newfoundland Hotel. We socialized together because we didn't really know anybody else. I met my future husband there. I didn't know then that he was going to be my husband, but we went to a party and I started going out with him. Several of us met our husbands in the same place. My friend and

I stayed for the four months and we went back but she didn't come back. I came back after a month because they allowed us to renew out visa for another six months.

"When I came back I worked again in the OR, but after I got married my husband got his first teaching job in Deer Lake so we moved there. I had culture shock when I came to St. John's, but when I went to Deer Lake I thought, 'Oh get me back to St. John's!' We moved there in January '75 and the snow was absolutely incredible. The west coast gets so much more snow. But we didn't ski because I went to work at Western Memorial in the recovery room for seven months.

"Then we went to England the following year because he hadn't met my family. My mom was the only one that came over for the wedding. I regret that now and wish I had done it differently, but my visa was about to expire and if I married a Canadian that automatically gave me landed immigrant status. But that wasn't the only reason why we got married! At the end of the seven months I was pregnant, so I quit working for three years because I had two children really close together in Corner Brook. I learned how to make bread, which I never thought I would, and various crafts and things. After three years I had enough of Deer Lake and thought 'This is it.'

"I had no problems understanding people, but there are some very strong accents around Howley. Deer Lake is quite different too ... I did have a bit of difficulty with the dialect. We were back and forth to England for the first three years of our marriage because my husband was writing his thesis in the second or third year of marriage. He said for me to take them home while he was doing that and I went for three months. When I returned I said, 'I want to move back to St. John's if we can. I don't want to stay out here.' He had gotten a chance of a job here at Brother Rice High School as a guidance counselor for a year. I said, 'Take it! If you don't take it I'm going home.' It ended up as a permanent position.

"When we came back, the children were two and three so I decided to work. By then I had written the RN exam for obstetrics, passed and got my RN. I did some casual shifts at St. Clare's and two of the shifts were terrible. I worked on the orthopedic unit and either evenings or nights were the only shifts I could work with small children and my husband a teacher. It was so hard and I didn't know the drugs. And the nurses weren't very welcoming. I got all the really bad assignments because I was only casual and they didn't know me. I used to cry every time I came home; I hated it. I did about three shifts when a good friend of mine, who was working at the Janeway, told me they were looking for nurses. She said, 'Put in an application,' which I did and got an interview. Then I got some casual work in the Emergency department there and loved it. It was like a big family at the Janeway and the nurses were really nice. I applied to work permanent but the only position they had was on the orthopedic ward. I took that, then asked for a transfer to emergency and got it within six months, and that's where I worked for the next 20 years.

"I didn't have any problems switching to pediatrics. It took a while to get the pediatric dosages but they were fabulous there. I got a good orientation. The head nurse was excellent, what a good nurse she was. I fit in with the Newfoundland nurses.

"When I left the Janeway, I went to work in the Poison Control Centre on the telephone advice line for four years and then to the recovery room for six months. Then I got a job at St. Clare's in the pre-admission because there was no shift work. It was eight-hour days, Monday to Friday. It was difficult moving from pediatrics to adults, even though I had done it years ago, because the drugs were different and I had to remember the adult diseases and medical problems. We had six weeks orientation at St. Clare's but it takes a good year to actually settle in. I've been there four years and I like it. It's busy.

"The challenge coming to Newfoundland was the big change in the culture. I came from a big city with lots to do, places to go and good shopping. I came here to St. John's and there was nothing. It was a shock but I thought for four months, I could do anything. But we had a good time and got to know lots of nice people who came over with us. Most of them went back unfortunately. It was an adventure. Never ever in my dreams did I think I would not go back to England. I went for holidays but not as often as I wanted, when the children were growing up, because I have four. It was too expensive.

"I found the people very friendly and helpful, other than that St. Clare's period, but I'm sure that wouldn't have lasted. Nurses are our own worst enemies sometimes. We're not always very welcoming. Other than that, the medications and procedures were different. Also the doctors had their own very different way of doing things and you had to know what they wanted. They put the fear into you, especially in the OR. They liked to be the be-all and end-all. That was their status. To them, the nurses were down here and the doctors were up there. It was the same in England but I don't think quite as much. I think it was worse here because I was in a different country and wasn't used to it.

"I wanted to be a nurse since I was 10 because of the uniform and no other reason. You were someone. Then I wore greens in the OR, which was a switch! Once I got into nursing I loved it. I've been in Newfoundland 33 years. We had our anniversary and one of the girls who came to Newfoundland with me came in. Another girl who came over with us phoned me when it was 30 years and said, 'Happy Anniversary.' I said to her, 'It's not my anniversary,' but she said 'Yes, it's June 2. We've been here 30 years.' I couldn't believe it! Usually the three of us get together. We all got married and stayed.

"One story stands out in my mind was when I was dating my husband. The cars were big back then and I wasn't used to driving on the right side of the road. My husband's friend had a big car with power steering and power brakes, and I wasn't used to those either. I had an international licence. I was driving his car and pulled up to the lights on Elizabeth Avenue but didn't realize that I should pump the brakes. The car didn't stop when it was supposed to and there was a young boy on a bike at the lights. Very slowly the car chewed up the back wheel of his bike. The boy looked around and said, 'What are you doing, lady?' I got out of the car and said, 'I'm so sorry. I didn't mean it.' He kept saying, 'Look at my bike! Look at my bike!' I drove him home and took him in. I rang the doorbell and out comes his father as stern as anything, and who was it but one of the doctors I worked with in the OR! I told him what happened, but he didn't say anything, just 'Very good.' I think he called me Nurse Brown because my name was Brown then. I was so frightened about going back to work, I wrote him a letter telling him what happened. He said he would send me a bill, but he didn't. I went to work absolutely terrified, but he never made any mention of it again.

"Another thing that really stands out is the snow. We had friends in Outer Cove and we could build tunnels going into their houses, there was so much snow. I've never gotten used to the winter and I still hate it. I always thought I'd go back to England at some point but each time I go now I like to come back here because I've spent more time in Newfoundland now than I did in England."

❀

Josephine (nee Brown) Hennebury was born in Lancaster, England. She graduated in 1972 as a SRN from Hope Hospital in Salford, England. She completed Part 1 midwifery at Stepping Hill Hospital in Stockport, Cheshire. In 1974 she immigrated to work at the St. John's General Hospital.

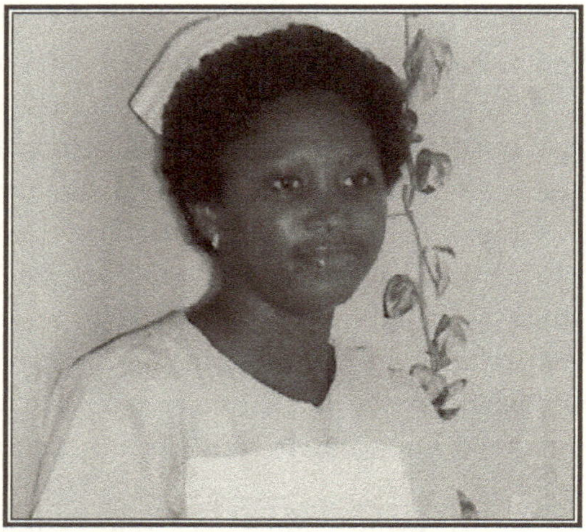

ERNESTINE (HARLESTON) WORLEY

2000

"I find life in Newfoundland okay. It is peaceful. I came from a war-torn country and I'm looking for peace. I have children going to school and Newfoundland is a good place to raise my kids."

"The nursing education system in Sierra Leone was exactly like the British system. After I graduated I practiced until I came here. I worked in general surgery, obstetrics and gynecology, and medicine. You weren't employed for a particular area. Then I worked in a military hospital for 14 and a half years in Freetown and went around the country to field hospitals and to the base hospital in the city. We were given the basic six months' training on how to parade and how to defend ourselves. We treated the soldiers.

"There were insurgencies from another country spilling over to Sierra Leone and I was a refugee in a neighbouring country with my family. The Canadian and United States governments identified certain refugees and said we were coming to Newfoundland. I didn't know where Newfoundland was. I thought it was a 'new found land!' We were resettled here in 2000. It was difficult moving and I had to adjust to the changes. There was a big difference in the two countries climate-wise. It was a total cultural shock. The winter of 2000 was a hard winter. My country has a tropical climate with a dry season and a rainy season. It's very hot. Totally different than Newfoundland!

"Sierra Leone is a British colony so we ate mostly what people eat here. The only difference we found was that we couldn't find a lot of different vegetables. Apart from that it wasn't so bad. We were received by the Association of New Canadians who gave us some orientation. We were taken around the city and shown where the supermarkets were. We were given a family doctor and were looked after by immigration. They would have supported us for a year, but I got a job in six months. We've had no problems fitting into the system.

"We got here on a Thursday and I went to church on a Sunday. I met a lady who asked me where was home and what was my profession? I told her and she gave me the telephone number for the ARNNL and I called them. I explained my situation and they gave me some forms to fill out. They wrote my college back home and it took about four months to get clarification of my documents. I was told to find a job and they would give me a temporary licence. I applied to the Health-care Corporation and they offered me a job with the surgery program. Then I wrote my board exam and passed.

"I've been at St. Clare's now for six and a half years. It's different practicing nursing here. I suppose it's like anywhere you go, the policies and procedures are different and in the surgical sections some of the equipment, like the pleurivac system, was new for me. At home we used the underwater chest tubes. Also certain drains like the

Hemovac drain and the Jackson-Pratt were new for me, but I found it was all the same nursing.

"I was given a two-week orientation because I hadn't practiced in Newfoundland before and I was grateful for that. I would have been more grateful for the six weeks! I worked on surgery and the girls on the floor were great. It took me about three months to find my footing. I was accepted by the other nurses. Initially it was difficult for them to understand me because the accent is different, but as time went by they understood me more and it rested solely on me accepting them. I believe that everywhere you go, if you love people they will return the same love to you, so that's what I practice. I understood the nurses' English but not some of the patients. If they were not wearing their dentures it was very difficult for me to understand what they were saying.

"The patients are curious about me. They want to know where I come from. That's the first thing they ask me, 'Where are you from?' And depending on who it is I'll tell them, 'I'm from Bell Island,' and I get them laughing before I tell them where I'm really from. They're not mean or nasty except when they're confused, and if they are confused you know how to deal with it. Sometimes when I go to work in the morning I ask God to give me patience, integrity, compassion and kindness and I go along with that.

"I find life in Newfoundland okay. It is peaceful. I haven't been home since I got here. My dad is still there, but they had an election and they had to leave the country because they were scared. They were going to be killed so it's still not settled there yet. I came from a war-torn country and I'm looking for peace. I have children going to school and Newfoundland is a good place to raise my kids. The last one is in university now and I don't think I could ask for anything more.

"I have practiced nursing for 26 years. Back home in Sierra Leone if you're a nurse or a teacher, you don't go into the profession for the money because you don't get paid much; you go into it because you love the job. I haven't regretted it. I love nursing.

"I registered some years ago for the BN (Post RN) program and I didn't do too badly. I'll continue with those courses some time."

�֎

Ernestine (nee Harleston) Worley was born in Freetown, Sierra Leone, in West Africa. She graduated in 1981 from the National School of Nursing in Freetown as an SRN. In 1983 she completed a one-year mid-wifery program (SCM) also in Freetown. Ernestine and her family came to Newfoundland and Labrador in 2000 as refugees from Gambia.

Section Two

IMMIGRATING TO NORTHERN NEWFOUNDLAND
AND COASTAL LABRADOR

Introduction

RECRUITMENT BY THE INTERNATIONAL GRENFELL ASSOCIATION FOR NORTHERN NEWFOUNDLAND AND COASTAL LABRADOR

OVERSEAS RECRUITMENT OF NURSES to Newfoundland and Labrador began when Wilfred Grenfell came to Labrador in 1892 to investigate living conditions among local fishers for the United Kingdom's National Mission to Deep Sea Fishermen. Shocked by the almost complete absence of health care services, Grenfell took it upon himself to raise money to establish regular health care services in Labrador and created the Grenfell Mission, later known as the International Grenfell Association (IGA). In 1893 Grenfell returned to Labrador with two doctors and two nurses to open a hospital in Battle Harbour.

Over time, Grenfell recruited volunteers and all categories of health care workers for IGA's health centres and funded IGA's work by lecturing about Labrador and accepting donations from wealthy individuals in the UK and the United States. This type of funding could not sustain the increasing cost of health care delivery and by the late 1970s, the Newfoundland and Labrador government subsidized the majority of funding for IGA facilities. In 1981, IGA turned over all its medical services to the government for $1.00 (J. Higgins, "Grenfell Mission: Newfoundland and Labrador Heritage"<www.heritage.nf.ca/society/grenfellmission> 2008).

Overseas recruitment for IGA differed from that in other areas of the province. IGA health facilities relied heavily on overseas nurses to supplement their workforce. They maintained an office in London to recruit all categories of health care workers and every effort was made to facilitate the immigration process for individuals.

Scott Smith worked in HR with IGA, and Aruna Thampy worked in Administration. Both were involved in recruitment of nurses and midwives for the northern region of the province, which originally encompassed the Labrador Coast, St. Anthony, and all nursing stations within the region, including Nain and Labrador down through to Harbour Deep, until the geographical boundaries of their health care facilities changed with restructuring. Both shared the IGA approach to recruitment and the related challenges.

RECRUITMENT

Scott Smith: "Until it shut in 1980, IGA had an office in the UK, run by a lady who was my contact person. She did our advertising and followed up on things like references. She'd contact us with suitable candidates, but we seldom said no because we were always short. She made the travel arrangements to Newfoundland and we met them here. After 1980, we used the office of a dentist we knew in the UK, rather than have the expense of our own. We'd advertise the position; the applications went to his office and his secretary sent them to us. We followed up the applications, references, and made appointments. When we were desperate we did the same with a doctor we knew in Ireland. One of the nurses and I then went to the UK and did interviews in a hotel. We did that two or three times and it worked out well; we brought back a lot of nurses. We recruited nurses from wherever we could get them; the Philippines, Australia, Nigeria, South Africa and New Zealand."

Aruna Thampy: "There was a never-ending need for nurses for the Labrador coast. We also recruited them for the directors in the hospital unless they came with us, but for the most part they left it to us. Twice a year we arranged career days in various schools and HR arranged recruiting sessions with schools of nursing on the mainland. They had little success with nursing schools in St. John's and Western. We visited the graduating classes and talked about coming to work with us. We spoke about nursing, especially on the coast, and HR talked about benefits and the environment. One disadvantage was we couldn't hire them for the nursing stations but did tell them they could go to a nursing station once they got experience.

"We agreed from the beginning that if we told the truth about the living conditions in the stations and they came, then they would stay. If someone was coming to a one-nurse station, we told them what it was like but also that we were moving to only two-nurse stations. We also had nurses who agreed to come after speaking to the station nurse. Nurses going to one-nurse stations had to have midwifery. We tried to get nurses with knowledge of pediatrics and mental health, but if they didn't have it and had issues, they could medevac the patient out. One of the nursing directors involved in recruiting would say, 'I know just the place for her. She would go well with ...' which speaks to the importance of having a nurse as part of recruitment.

"Travelling to England to recruit for IGA started in the 1980s and '90s because we were strapped for nurses. We prepared brochures: about the nursing stations, the populations, and what the communities were like. We had a package of information along with pictures and a video of Curtis Memorial [the hospital in St. Anthony], the area, and the people. I oversaw what was sent out. But by then we realized that recruiting simply on kindness, snowshoeing, and skiing, and showing a beautiful video wasn't going to get them to come anymore. Also we were recruiting more Canadians nurses and skiing wasn't a privilege for them. So we had to look at what could we offer them. But we got more sophisticated as we went to job fairs and saw what other people had.

"You always had to be on top of the game when recruiting and we were persistent. If we recruited a nurse from Australia and she called to speak to the director of nursing we treated that seriously. With the different time zones I'd get up at 2:00 a.m. to return that call because she might get a call from somebody else and we'd lose that window of opportunity. If they said, 'I'll only come for a year,' we never said anything. When they got used to the place and started to enjoy it, then we started our recruitment and retention strategy."

Scott Smith: "We never had the situation where we had too many nurses. There were times when there were unemployed nurses in Canada and we were at risk of having to dismiss some of the overseas nurses to hire them. Some years back there was an abundance of nurses in St. John's and unemployed nurses were calling the Newfoundland Hospital Association saying, 'We can't get work and we're going to leave.' I had advised the hospital association that we had no nurses and they told them to call me in St. Anthony. I'd get them a job, but their answer was always, 'I don't want to go up there.'"

INCENTIVES

Scott Smith: "Initially when we recruited in the UK, our salaries were much better. Then salaries in the UK went above ours so that wasn't an incentive any longer."

Aruna Thampy: "We didn't offer much except friendship and support and told them what a wonderful place Newfoundland was. We talked about the adventure and challenges of working on the coast, if that was what they were looking for. One of the nursing directors mothered the nurses like when they came to St. Anthony she invited them to her home. Non-monetary things like kindness worked well with the nurses we recruited. If the *Beaver* was going to a station and the nurses were dying for fruit and vegetables, she'd buy it and send it on the flight. In my view it was those things that kept nurses on the coast. It had nothing to do with money."

ACCOMMODATIONS

Scott Smith: "IGA had accommodations, which helped. Nurses got a subsidized rate so it was relatively inexpensive to come and work for us. In St. Anthony they had one- or two-bedroom heated apartments, which was better than any accommodations they could afford in London. One downfall was that sometimes the nurses had to share with someone they didn't know, but for others it was a positive because they met people and got involved in the community much faster."

Aruna Thampy: "The nurses had the comfort of knowing when they arrived we would look after them. Everything was subsidized on the coast. If you lived in a nursing station your room and meals were provided. At one time we had cooks but they went when budgets got tight. The nurses had to take care of themselves, which worried me because I thought they needed to be looked after especially when they did clinics all day, but the nurses adapted. The newer nurses didn't want a cook. They wanted to cook for themselves.

"We didn't pay for a nurse to bring her husband; he paid his own way, and nurses who came with families had to rent their own apartments in St. Anthony, although rents were reasonable in those days. However, they paid the way out for a doctor and his family and subsidized their houses in St. Anthony."

ORIENTATION

Scott Smith: "Having things in place to help them adapt was not one of our strongest points. A nurse met them when they arrived and took them to their apartment. We had a welcome bag in their apartment so they didn't have to rush out for milk and juice or whatever. In the early days our aircraft picked them up in Gander and brought them to St. Anthony.

"The day after they arrived we did the necessary paperwork and I told them how to reach me if they had any problems or issues. They had a one-week to two-week orientation to meet various people. We took them around the community, especially in St. Anthony and showed them the bank, the grocery store, and the churches and anything else they needed to know.

"Nurses going to the stations had a much longer orientation. They met with the doctors who would be their lifeline by telephone. Initially they did that through the RT .... In later years, the nurse came in and met the physicians and lab staff because these were the people they were dependent on. It wasn't uncommon for some nurses to have extensive orientation periods. Nursing services assessed them to determine their weak points. If they went to a clinic and were not strong in some areas they came back to St. Anthony for further orientation. Some were exceptionally good, and caught on really fast, probably due to experience, but others either weren't fast or were more reserved.

"We always encouraged the nurses working in St. Anthony to get experience and see the types of patients the station nurses sent into the hospital. We gave them an opportunity to observe that and we made arrangements for them to go to a station and shadow a nurse for a weekend or on their days off, if they wanted, to see if they liked it. But not everyone was cut out for that. If they didn't like the nursing stations they could get one or two years' experience at the hospital and go to a station if they wanted to."

IMMIGRATION CHALLENGES

Scott Smith: "Canada Employment and ARNNL were some of the challenges we encountered. One of the biggest was how slow things happened with immigration. We had to do a job search in Canada because we always had a standing order for nurses in Canada. We did what we had to do on this end before we placed an ad. Once we secured a nurse in the UK, we did the necessary paperwork within a day or so and sent it to the Human Resources Canada Centre. We had an office in St. Anthony so things weren't too bad, and Immigration in Gander was pretty good because they knew our needs. They'd have a turnaround time of two to three weeks and we'd have the paperwork back with their approval. That went to the Canadian consulate office in London or Dublin or Edinburgh, depending on where the nurse came from. There it went into a file for sometimes three or four months before it was processed. The nurse had to get a medical, a criminal search, and things like that. Sometimes the file was delayed so long I had to get on the telephone to the Immigration Department in Canada to see if they could put pressure on the UK people. I even went to politicians in Ottawa and said, 'We need to get this nurse here. We're trying to provide health care. What can you do?' Sometimes that worked. We only did that when we were desperate. Sometimes we lost a nurse because it took so long getting things processed.

"Grenfell also sponsored anybody who wanted to come as landed immigrants. It was more complex if a nurse wanted landed immigrant status. That meant she had to stay in England longer and we couldn't afford that wait. We did whatever we could to assist them, but the biggest thing was a job offer because so many points were given for a job."

Aruna Thampy: "Most of ours came on temporary permits until the Government of Canada made it easier. We were only allowed to bring a nurse over if we couldn't get a Canadian nurse, so we had to provide justification that we couldn't get a Canadian nurse, but we never had any problem justifying for the coast. The Immigration Department was very good working with us, particularly with station nurses and with hospital nurses. Sometimes, if there were difficulties and delays, the Director of Nursing, or somebody in HR or the CEO, would call Immigration. They were slower with hospitals and always asked, 'Why can't you get a Canadian nurse?'"

ARNNL CHALLENGES

Aruna Thampy: "We got permission from ARNNL to bring nurses in on temporary licences because it took so long. They weren't paid a registered nurse salary until they wrote the RN exams. If they came on temporary licences they stayed at St. Anthony hospital where they were safe, because we had to make sure they were safe. If they were experienced nurses they went to a nursing station, but we had to give them time to study and they didn't always get that time in the station."

"Grenfell always wanted the nurse yesterday. I think after a while that really grated on the people at ARNNL and they'd ask, 'What are you people doing?' The thing was that we never knew when somebody was leaving. The registrar at the association has a clear mandate, which I didn't understand but then I never asked. I don't think St. John's really understood how we worked in the north and we felt they didn't care about us. We thought, 'Who are these people bugging us?' If there was a problem with ARNNL, we paid the registration fee and the nurse reimbursed us. It was quicker! We found loopholes—a way to make it happen. I think that sometimes annoyed the registering body even more."

Scott Smith: "Some nurses were distraught and disappointed having to write the RN exam. Most provincial hospitals paid them as unregistered nurses until they got registered. When they passed the registration exams we paid them retroactive to their commencement date. I don't know if that was an incentive, but they knew what their salary would be once they passed the exams and had money coming to them. Some didn't want to write registration exams when they came, but we always reassured them they would pass and that we would pay them retroactively."

Nurses recruited by IGA worked either in one of the IGA's hospitals, clinics, or a nursing station on the Labrador coast. The majority of these nurses trained in large teaching hospitals in London. If posted to a nursing station, the nurses could be required to work alone in isolated communities where they encountered situations for which their training programs did not prepare them. Not surprisingly these nurses had to make significant adjustments to the working environment, in their practice, and in their lifestyle. However, as the sole health care provider, the nurse was often embraced by the community.

A nurse stationed at the hospital in St. Anthony found a different set of circumstances. A large number of the hospital nursing staff was British-trained, so newly-recruited nurses found that they came into a medical community where many of the practices and routines were based on what they knew. Many of the staff at St. Anthony came from similar education and work backgrounds and understood the needs of the new nurse. Newcomers were included in social activities and staff helped them to get settled and become familiar with the community and local services. Nurses coming to St. Anthony essentially joined a community of other immigrant health care workers who worked with IGA.

Scott Smith: "Recruitment of nurses is a continuous effort because now the only place we can get nurse midwives is the UK, but in the last few years that supply was drying up. We wouldn't have been able to operate without the nurse midwives. There were times when we didn't have an obstetrician gynecologist on staff and the midwives were invaluable. Even if we have obstetrician gynecologists today, they can't work 24/7. The midwifery aspect was invaluable especially in the smaller areas and the experienced nurses in the outpost nursing stations were worth their weight in gold."

Nurses working in northern Newfoundland and on the Labrador coast encountered working technologies and methods not common to health care delivery. For many years their primary means of communicating was the RT, which was how nurses in the stations and clinics talked to St. Anthony and vice versa. There was a 'sched' as required. This was a *scheduled* call for nurses in the stations to discuss cases with a doctor and to talk to nurses in the clinics, and whether they got through or not depended on the atmospheric conditions at the time. The job of the RT operator on duty was to listen for emergency calls and send things to communities that were needed, like medications. Also it was usually the first point of contact for nurses arriving in the province.

The primary transportation method was small float planes or Beaver planes or helicopter. These were used to transport or 'medevac' patients from their community to hospital, particularly in emergency situations.

This section focuses on the experiences of nurses who worked with IGA in northern Newfoundland and coastal Labrador and is divided into three groups: nurses who worked in the nursing stations, those who worked in IGA-operated hospitals, and those recruited specifically as nurse midwives for St. Anthony, where they can legally practice in the province. It was not uncommon for nurses to move between hospitals and nursing stations within IGA facilities, sometimes by choice but more often in response to need.

These nurses' stories provide insight into health care delivery in areas serviced by IGA, socio-economic circumstances in northern and coastal communities, along with the unbelievable challenges they encountered. As with other nurses we have interviewed, this group did what they had to do, often under extremely difficult circumstances. In many cases they were the sole health care provider to the people of northern Newfoundland and coastal Labrador but accepted the responsibility of primary caregiver and advocate for the people they served.

Chapter Four

COASTAL LABRADOR

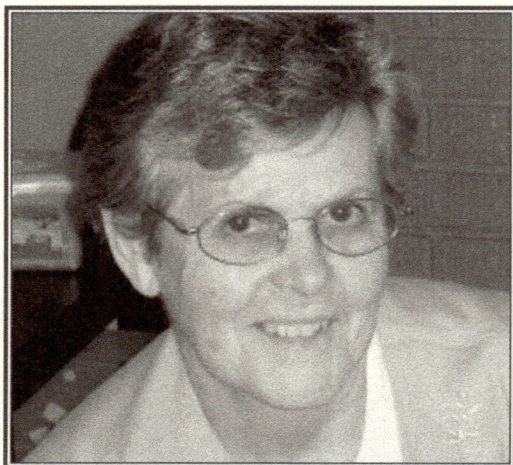

ISOBEL (ROBINSON) WATTS

❁

1961

"The children stand out most for me because they had daily streptomycin injections and were so brave and stoic—braver than adults taking needles!"

"I did midwifery because I wanted to travel and midwifery was pretty mandatory. A Grenfell doctor visited my brother's boarding school to talk about Grenfell. He sent me the information on IGA in a Grenfell Christmas card and it stuck in my imagination. I wrote to the IGA in London, who were very keen to get staff, and was interviewed by someone at their London office. I had good references and they depended on those. I came to North West River hospital straight from finishing midwifery training and was surprised I could go so soon because I thought they'd need people with lots of experience.

"I came to work in North West River but they were short a nurse in Happy Valley, so I spent time there and then went back and forth between North West River and Happy Valley. Eventually they got a nurse in Happy Valley, but she didn't like it so we changed every week. Finally she stayed in Happy Valley and I stayed in North West River.

"I came to Goose Bay via Gander in June. It was so different! They met me at the airport in a vehicle called Willie's truck and we drove to Goose River. Some boys were coming home from school in St. John's and I couldn't understand a word they were saying. I don't think they understood me either, although we all spoke English. We crossed the river in a boat and there was another truck on the other side. We drove to North West River then took a canoe across to the hospital. There were no bridges then, we didn't even have the cable car.

"I didn't dress in high fashion but here I was in my little English suit and shoes with my suitcase. Someone pointed in the direction of the hospital and said, 'Just walk up the wharf and onto the path and the hospital is right there.' I opened the hospital door and a young man rushed past me down the path. It was the doctor going to meet me! The outpatients' clinic was near the entrance and someone said, 'The nurses are upstairs.' I met the head nurse, who was also British. I was the third nurse. They tried to have three nurses but usually there were only two, which was hard.

"My worst challenge was understanding the people because they pronounced some words differently. It wasn't bad face-to-face, but I had a hard time on the telephone sometimes!

"The hospital in North West River was well-equipped and up to date, which surprised me. The only bad thing was the lab. The doctors did as much lab work as they could, but we sent a lot to St. John's. That wasn't a good system because it got broken or lost in the mail. But we survived.

"Working in North West River was straightforward because people had their schedules and the system was running well, so I joined the team and got on with it. The hospital had about 40 beds, which weren't always full. There were about 10 aides whom we trained along with the maids, three to four doctors and three nurses on staff. The doctors were British and came for a year. I came for two years, but at the end I was the only registered nurse on staff. We had a female doctor who did some nursing jobs because I couldn't do it alone. Then we got a second and third nurse. That was 1963. I collapsed twice that year with an aneurism. The first time they weren't sure and sent me to Montreal for a rest. But I collapsed again on Boxing Day and was rushed back to Montreal to have a clip put in. Meanwhile I had gotten engaged but we hadn't told anybody. When I came back, the doctor asked me to stay as head nurse so I told him I was getting married. We married in England.

"There was a lot of TB in those days. Adults from the coast went to St. Anthony. Most of the children with TB stayed with us unless they were really bad. They were in two rooms. Most came from the Inuit communities. It was sad because they were in hospital for six months and never saw their parents. We had someone on staff from England who did activities with them and kept them happy. The children stand out most for me because they had daily streptomycin injections and were so brave and stoic—braver than adults taking needles! Quite a few are still in Sheshatshiu and are healthy now. There's TB around again but we did a good job of getting rid of most of it. It's wonderful to see the improvement in medical care here. I remember one year when every baby born on the coast of Labrador died.

"We had no seniors' home here and those who were bedridden, with no one at home to care for them, took up beds. They'd be in at least a year and required a lot of nursing care, but we were young and strong. The aides helped and knew the language. Others stayed until they died because there was nowhere else to go. Later they sent them to St. John's or somewhere. We also had four obstetric beds and an isolette for preemies. I worked as a midwife because we had a lot of obstetrics. We delivered babies in the clinic, we didn't do home deliveries.

"I was amazed by the stoic nature of the natives. They didn't fuss about anything. Take child delivery: some didn't make a sound, they were silent. People in North West River are of Scottish extraction, but they're mixed, Scottish and Inuit. My husband is counted as Inuit because his mother was born in Lake Melville and his father was from Brigus. Everyone in North West River spoke English. The coastal Inuit mostly spoke English, but the Innu had their own language and sometimes we needed an interpreter.

"North West River was the main hospital for the region. A plane was based there and picked up patients in coastal communities from Cartwright and north. We also did clinics in the communities. I went to Rigolet a few times because there was no nurse or doctor there. We checked the school children's heads, which was a chore. I helped the doctor do tooth extractions because there was no dentist. When I was relieving in Nain, I pulled a fellow's tooth. The poor chap was desperate! I also relieved in Makkovik. We went in to give the nurse a rest because some clinics had only one nurse. A dentist visited the communities once a year and an eye specialist came from England to do clinics once a year. Otherwise, if the people needed a doctor they had to come to North West River.

"Relieving in the stations was pretty routine because the staff knew what they were doing. We just did clinics and delivered babies. One night in Nain I got a call, and if somebody called, you were expected to visit. You didn't tell them to come to the hospital in the middle of the night. The funny thing was that I had a temperature of 102 Fahrenheit but was feeling all right so I hiked to the end of the village to see a lady with pins and needles in her arms. That's all that was wrong with her! I said, 'If they're still there tomorrow, come to the hospital.' On my way back a dog, which I thought was a wolf, followed me to the clinic.

"They had a lot of huskies, and while I was there we inoculated 900 dogs with distemper vaccine. We worked with the Mounties and the nurses' aide. People had maybe 10 or 12 dogs in a team and they'd hold them for us. We'd draw up about 10 ccs of vaccine and give one cc at a time before it froze. It was very cold but it was fun. One of the doctors operated on the animals because there was no vet. We also did some veterinary work like anesthetizing the dogs and cats!

"I probably visited every community on the coast helping with clinics or picking up patients. I went to Grand Lake to find an Innu camp where the people were camped. We got a message saying they needed someone, so we went by float plane to the head of Grand Lake and finally saw smoke rising from the camp. It was a very sick child who had flu and her head was covered with impetigo that was crusted over.

"I spent time in Happy Valley, which had about 6,000 people at the time. The nursing station had four beds. It was supposed to have two nurses and a doctor but they were so short staffed I filled in. There was also a lot of obstetrics there. We sent overnight patients to North West River's hospital, but if we kept patients we had to cook. I didn't think I should have to because I wasn't very good. They hired a cook, but if the cook wasn't there we took turns cooking! I preferred North West River because it was mostly in-patients and had an OR, whereas Happy Valley was mostly outpatients and babies.

"The nurses were a great bunch, although I didn't get to know them really well. I keep in touch with most of the people I worked with. I correspond with a girl I worked with in Happy Valley who is in England and a head nurse who is in Scotland. Whenever I go home I try to see them, but they're scattered all over the place.

"After I married I worked part-time at the Springdale cottage hospital, but not for long because I had babies. I went wherever my husband's work took him. When we were in North West River I did Red Cross Clinics and some volunteer work. I also did immunizations and some baby work because there was no public health nurse. We visited the Innu people in their homes or tents across the river, because they wouldn't come to clinics. After a delivery we wanted to be sure everything was all right, so we'd take their blood pressures and that kind of thing. We also visited and treated the old people in their homes and that was interesting. We had an interpreter paid by the hospital.

"We came back to North West River because of my husband's work. There are about 550 people here. We have two sons and we're grandparents of a boy and girl. When I worked, my relatives didn't visit, but my brother and father visited us in Springdale and here also. I worked full-time for two and a half years after I came, but then was off with this sickness business. I would have gone back if I'd been in the right place at the right time but nothing clicked. I got involved in the community doing volunteer work. I did arts and crafts, have been involved with music in the community, helped out with art at the school and am in charge of a volunteer library. These things helped throughout my life and I'm never bored.

"I loved nursing in Labrador; I really did! I was devastated when I had to leave it. There were sad times. I remember one baby who just suffocated with pneumonia. I was 24 when I came and it was a lot of responsibility for someone. When I look back I think, 'My goodness!'"

❈

Isobel (nee Robinson) Watts was born near Gainford, England. She graduated in 1958 as a SRN from the Nightingale School of Nursing at St. Thomas's Hospital in London. She completed midwifery as a SCM at Freedom Fields Hospital in Plymouth in 1961 before immigrating to work at the North West River nursing station that same year.

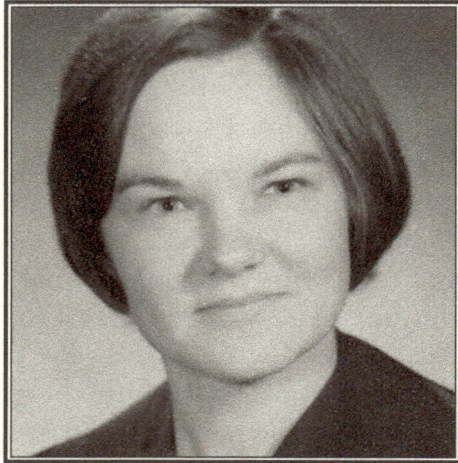

ANNE CHAULK

✳

1961

*"The Newfoundland community was new to me and I liked
the community aspect. We had to make our own entertainment,
which I enjoyed, along with getting to know people."*

"Around graduation my friend and I were looking for another job so we
decided to come to Canada. We didn't know how to apply or have
much information and thought we'd have to come by boat. My friend
met some medical students who had worked with IGA. They told us
about it and put us in touch with the recruiting person for IGA in
London. It was as simple as that! They had the forms we had to
complete there and they helped us with the formalities and procedures.

"When I arrived in Gander I thought, 'These people speak English but I can't understand a word they're saying.' I barely remember Gander but it was very emotional because I had just left England and wondered what I was coming to. I came in March but my friend wasn't free to come for another month. She was recruited for St. Anthony and I went to North West River. When I got there it looked like pictures I had seen. I came for a year and stayed because I was enjoying myself.

"There were lots of challenges in nursing because things were very different from London. North West River was a cottage hospital with four or five nurses who came and went. I travelled occasionally to relieve in the nursing stations on the coast. That was one of our duties and I wanted to do it. We relieved for a month to six weeks in each station while the permanent nurse had a vacation. The coastal communities were tiny and there was a lot of TB. We were on call 24 hours a day, which was exhausting, especially at the busiest stations because the communities were new to me and I knew very few people. We did home visits similar to what we did in England except there were the Aboriginal cultures.

"When I arrived in North West River things were changing. They had introduced an eight-hour shift system into the hospital, which was what I was used to in London. The year before I arrived, nurses did split shifts where they went to work at seven or eight in the morning, got two or three hours off in the afternoon and went back to work until eight at night. I worked them in Maine and they were tiring because you did nothing, only work—and in your two hours off you slept.

"First when I came, Canadian nurses at the hospital took each summer off and still had a job when they came back. They went on vacation for however long they wanted and only two of us were left. We'd worked 12-hour night shifts for 10 days to two weeks without a break, because we had to be there for surgery or if anything happened. The other nurse did days and I did nights. It was tiring! We were supposed to get a couple of weeks' vacation but it seemed to go on forever. Our accommodations were provided so we slept in the hospital.

"We flew to the coast a lot in six-seat Beavers, which were the main method of transportation. We brought in patients who weren't really sick but needed a nurse to accompany them. They weren't like the medevacs of today because we rarely had ventilated patients. The planes landed on water or ice, which was very exciting for me! It was an adventure and I enjoyed it. We used a closed-in snowmobile to take patients from the hospital to the air strip. We also had little snow-mobiles which were a smaller version of what's available today.

"I was in charge of the smaller nursing stations but worked as a staff nurse in Melville and at the Labrador Health Centre. Melville was the old United States Air Force Hospital in Happy Valley which was sold to the provincial government when the Americans pulled out in the '70s. The hospital had a dedicated maternity area, which was quite different because it was isolated from the general area of the hospital. I've worked as a midwife for the last 20 years and still occasionally work at the Labrador Health Centre in Happy Valley-Goose Bay. Things have changed since the new hospital was built because maternity is integrated now and not nearly as midwifery-linked, but then they can't recruit midwives like they did.

"Life in North West River was busy but interesting. The culture was so different. It was a challenge and a change and I enjoyed it because it was so different. North West River was small but I came from a small village in England so I didn't mind that. The Newfoundland community was new to me and I liked the community aspect. We had to make our own entertainment, which I enjoyed along with getting to know people. We'd sit around chatting or have a sing-song or potluck meal. One of the girls rented a house and there was always a kitchen party going on which included the local people as well as the hospital people. People from the community would just drop in.

"I'm happy I became a nurse because nursing was an opportunity in my life and I got to travel. I go to London for vacation and have always kept in touch with my family. That was important to me because my parents supported my decision to stay here. They have visited because this is my home now."

❧

Anne Chaulk was born in Birmingham, England. She graduated from the Royal Free Hospital School of Nursing in London in 1965 as an SRN. She completed midwifery as a SCM in 1966 before immigrating to work at the North West River nursing station in 1967.

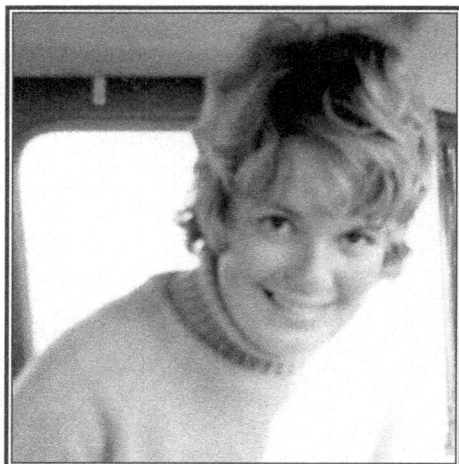

ISOBEL (MUIR) RUMBOLT

❈

1973

*"I was 25 when I came. If I knew then what I know now, I don't think
I'd have come. I had no idea of what I was getting into. You lived
day-to-day and didn't worry about things like you do when you're older."*

"I saw a job advertised in a nursing journal but midwifery was required.
My friend was also coming but hadn't done midwifery so I waited until
she did that and got some experience. My mother heard Dr. Grenfell
speak in a parish hall in Glasgow in the 1930s. I didn't know what to do
after I graduated and she thought I'd like Labrador.

"We were nervous and intimidated going to London for the
interview but when we walked in, the lady looked at us and said, 'When

can you go to Canada?' There was no interview process! I guess our references did it. We had to get immunizations, a passport, and a work permit, but Grenfell arranged that for us.

"My friend and I came to Gander where the hospital's little seven-seat plane picked us up. That was a shock! It was very cold and almost dark when we landed in St. Anthony. We worked at the hospital there for three months and lived in a very nice staff house. It was March and not too cold but lots of snow and so pretty. We thought we had died and gone to heaven!

"When we applied, there were jobs in St. Anthony, but after three months the supervisor of the nursing stations asked if we were interested in going to Labrador. The two nurses in Mary's Harbour were going to England for further training and their jobs were open for a year. I signed a one-year contract and this would extend my stay, but we agreed because we could go there together.

"It was a beautiful day when we landed in Mary's Harbour in the float plane, but it struck me as being so isolated from the air. The arctic drift ice was still around, which made it more spectacular. The nursing station was a beautiful building with in-patients. The nurses were leaving the next day so we had a one-day, 24-hour orientation. They tried to tell us everything in those 24 hours but also made a list for us to refer to. It was a terrible shock! At the end of that day, we looked at each other and said, 'What are we doing here? What have we gotten ourselves into?'

"We covered a large area with no road contact so we travelled either by plane, boat, or on Ski-Doo in the winter. The closest nurse to us was in Cartwright. There was no doctor so we worked similar to a GP. We had a system to call the doctors, who were excellent and a big support for us. We held daily clinics and one of us went to the other communities. It was scary though, because we didn't know what was coming through the door. Some communities didn't have a nurse, so we got a lot of telephone calls because we were their caregivers and had their charts.

"We called St. Anthony a lot! I probably called a doctor, especially the pediatrician, once or twice a day. We had a lot of sick kids with croup, bronchitis, skin infections, and bad ears. I wouldn't take a risk with children and many times we medevaced them to St. Anthony, but when they got there they weren't that bad. You just worried about them. Also if you got a phone call from Port Hope-Simpson or Charlottetown you couldn't see the patient. You listened to a distraught mother or an un-trained lay dispenser and you had to decide whether to get the mission plane or treat the child overnight and call in the morning. You had to deal with all sorts of variables, so we tended to err on the side of caution.

"Trying to diagnose illness on the telephone was the biggest challenge of all. We had lay dispensers in each community and the telephone was in their house. They had a drug box with certain drugs they could give with authority from the doctor in St. Anthony or, if we couldn't find a doctor, we prescribed something. They had narcotics for severe pain because they were so far away from us. Those ladies were good. They took temperatures and could give you a feel if someone was an emergency. They weren't trained but had a lot of common sense and were a wonderful support for us. They were volunteers and didn't get paid, so we gave them free drugs for their family and at Christmas we sent a hamper. It was a bartering thing, which was fine, and they were happy with that. We had first-aid kits with a few select drugs and things in each community because the weather could be bad for days on end, and there was no way of getting anything to them because the plane wasn't flying. The system worked well, but you couldn't do that nowadays with so many protocols and policies. People would freak out!

"Once a month or every six weeks in winter we did a Ski-Doo trip around the district. We had a guide who was paid to take us every day because we weren't allowed to travel on Ski-Doo or by boat alone. We bought his gas and he stayed with relatives or friends at our destination, but there was no money exchanged. We stayed with the lay dispensers and they fed us. They were a lifeline!

"It was nice to come with a friend, because in the nursing stations the nurse is all things to all people and you depend on each other. She and I had to agree on everything, from how much meat to order each week to whether we were going to treat a child. We had to get along because we were stressed a lot and being friends helped. Also our confidence wasn't great so we worked together in a buddy system and found that better. With only two of us at the station and our buddy system, we didn't get days off. We did get vacations because somebody from St. Anthony relieved. We tried to get a night's sleep every second night, but most nights we got a lot of phone calls at night and the station had 10 in-patient beds.

"We had nursing aides who were local girls. They took temperatures, kept fluid charts, and did basic nursing. One worked at night to look after the in-patients, but lots of times she had to wake us up. It was the magnitude of looking after other communities by phone, caring for in-patients, and having to do out-patient clinics.

"We were overworked and really earned our money. We had one or two deliveries a week and patients with strokes or chronic obstructive lung disease. We kept children for observation if we didn't know what was wrong, or if they had bronchitis or croup. Then we might have trauma. It was so varied! We did a lot of dental work, like simple extractions, and we weren't prepared for that. I did my first extraction when the dentist visited. He showed us what to do and told us what was beyond our capabilities. He visited every three months and a doctor came every two months. We had a referral list when he came. It was such a relief when the doctor came!

"Working in the hospital in Mary's Harbour was different. We had a lot of native patients from northern Labrador who didn't speak English very well. That was one of my biggest challenges. My accent was strongly Scottish and people here had a different accent. There were misunderstandings sometimes even though we all spoke English. Phrases and sayings were so different like 'She's got a wonderful pain!' That was confusing! My first patient in Mary's Harbour said, 'She had a pain in the pole.' Try to figure out where that is! Rural words like that were quite confusing!

"The first year was very intimidating until we got used to the way of life and different culture. Getting used to the different mealtimes was culture shock. Dinner in Scotland is called supper here, so when we were asked to dinner we didn't go in the middle of the day. When we appeared in the evening, they'd say, 'What are you doing here?' That happened several times until we got used to it. For me lunch was in the middle of the day, but here it's a snack in-between meals. We got things straightened out after a while. We relaxed a bit after the first year and started to enjoy things more.

"We had a whooping cough epidemic and bad influenza my first winter here. It wasn't a cold and runny nose thing; it was full-blown flu! A lot of children got whooping cough and if they weren't immunized they had it really bad. One baby died, but he was less than three weeks old and hadn't been immunized. Most were immunized, so although they were quite sick they got better. Every school in the district was closed for two weeks and we made extra trips to communities that didn't have a nurse. We'd take boxes of cough syrup and give out packs when we got there. Some older people developed pneumonia and some of the babies were quite sick. Another year we had four crib deaths in one winter, but you don't hear that sort of thing anymore. That was so sad. We'd get a call that a child was dead in the crib. If it was in our community, we'd rush over to a house but always be too late. But if it was in another community the mission plane went in to get the body.

"The two nurses we replaced decided not to return so we got permanent positions. I stayed another year then got married and travelled to different communities with my husband, who is a teacher. I've been in Labrador ever since.

"IGA opened a clinic in Port Hope Simpson and one in Charlotte-town, which helped us in Mary's Harbour enormously. It reduced having to diagnose by telephone and we didn't have in-patients. We went from nursing station to nursing clinic with only a holding bed in case we had to admit a patient until the plane came. We only kept someone if the weather was bad, which happened a lot. Our practice was very weather dependent!

"I went to Charlottetown clinic on my own, which took getting used to because there was nobody to talk things over with. It wasn't the same workload as Mary's Harbour and I was on call every night. The community had never had a resident nurse and was glad to have somebody. I was invited for meals and they'd call to see if I needed anything. Everyone was friendly and made me feel very welcome.

"Charlottetown had two satellite communities which were coastal fishing stations where people moved each summer. We travelled the coast on the hospital ship Strathcona and were considered one of the crew. We made three trips, which lasted a week every summer to 27 summer communities. There was no telephone on board, only the RT set which we used to contact people. There was an x-ray on board, a dental room, a room for the public health nurse, and one for the doctor. The doctor and I worked together. We took equipment, drugs, charts, and first-aid emergency stuff so we were prepared.

"We had a list of referrals and the skipper called out the names on the loudspeaker and the people came to the boat. It was a walk-in clinic type of thing. We gave medications to whoever needed them and treated people if they were sick. Our visit was an event because these were wee fishing communities with only three or four families. They would come to see what was happening. It was fun.

"Communications in the summer weren't very good. You might get a message via the RT or someone travelling from a community would bring a note. We had some funny notes. A man came for a blood pressure check and as he was leaving he said, 'By the way, nurse, I have a note for you.' All it said was, 'Nurse, come quick, my baby is sick.' We were always prepared to go and had everything ready in a closet. We packed it onto a komatik, which we travelled on in the winter. It had boxes on board and everything was always ready to go. You just had to grab the chart. I went back with him and the baby wasn't well; it had breathing problems. When I finished, the man brought me back. The people were just wonderful helping out in situations.

"After I married we went to Port Hope Simpson and I took a position there. One night a young man became very ill and was hemorrhaging badly. I called St. Anthony and from my description they didn't think he'd survive the night. They sent the mission plane and medevaced him to St. Anthony. That was the first time that happened because those planes fly visually. They didn't encourage flying at night but that was an emergency. The RT wanted all lights in the community turned off so the pilot could see the outline of the harbour and wharf to land the plane. They didn't send a nurse because we wanted as few people as possible on the plane when it landed in Port Hope Simpson. I flew back with the patient because it was brighter in St. Anthony and there'd be no problem landing there. The patient went to the OR immediately and survived. But that was a very anxious night!

"We moved to St. Lewis, but there wasn't a clinic there, so I worked in a private home in the community. We had a small room upstairs and the patients waited in the living room. I had cupboards built in the hall where I stored things. The people were paid for the use of their home, but it wasn't very much. Clinic was from 9:00 to 12:00 and 1:00 to 5:00, but things happened during the meal hour or at night, which was disturbing for the family. The house was always open so I didn't need a key, but I had keys for the upstairs room and the drug cupboards which were always locked. I resigned after my daughter was born and relieved the nurses in the area.

"My mom was interested when I came here because she'd heard of Dr. Grenfell. My dad wasn't so fussy and said afterwards that he knew when I got on the plane to Canada I would never come back to live. A father's intuition! They visited here before I married and again after I had children. They loved it because it's so much like the north of Scotland. It's more isolated and has less population, but the land is similar and fishing is the mainstay of the economy. There are a lot of similarities to Scotland. My father died but Mom has made many trips here, and I've gone to Scotland on vacation. People ask why I stay, but I enjoy the outdoors and you have to live here. There is beautiful scenery and boating, hiking, and skiing, and I do them all in moderation. I get on a Ski-Doo and have the freedom to travel over the hills, lakes, and ponds. It's so different from home.

"We were in St. Lewis for seven years, but I gave up after my fourth child because it was too hard. I really enjoyed working in the nursing stations. It was interesting and a great learning opportunity. I grew up fast because I had such responsibility. The good times certainly outweighed the bad. Being able to travel and get out of the clinic environment and into people's homes was good. We had wonderful support systems in place, like the plane and the doctors in St. Anthony who were so helpful to us on the telephone. Without those it would have been hard. Even though I was in the clinic on my own I knew I had people to rely on.

"I was 25 when I came. If I knew then what I know now, I don't think I'd have come. I had no idea of what I was getting into. You lived day-to-day and didn't worry about things like you do when you're older. I gave up 18 years ago after working 25 years. We moved back to Mary's Harbour about 20 years ago because my husband is from here and he returned to teaching here."

❋

Isobel (nee Muir) Rumbolt was born in Glasgow, Scotland. She graduated as a SRN from Western Infirmary in Glasgow, Scotland, in 1969. She completed a diploma in midwifery as a SCM in 1971 from the Glasgow Royal Maternity Hospital in Glasgow.

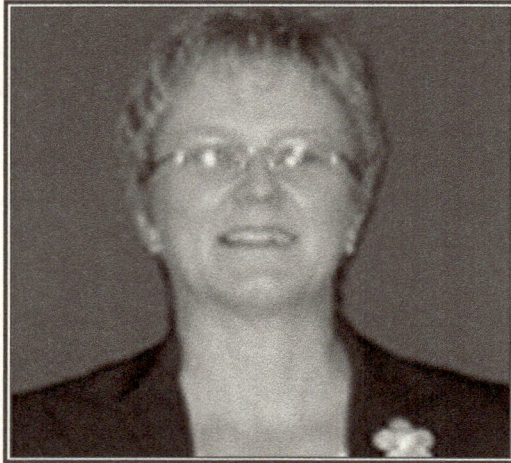

SUE (FROUDE) WEBB

❋

1975

"I've had the most amazing career anyone could wish for in Newfoundland and Labrador ... It's been a real experience, with highs and lows and challenges you wouldn't believe, but it's been fantastic."

"I had a job on the *QEII* but needed another year of experience in accident and emergency. I was looking for a one-year contract, but everywhere had only two-year contracts. My friend and I wanted to go overseas and I saw a little advert that said 'one-year contract.' I made enquiries and two of our obstetricians had been to Newfoundland with the IGA. I applied in October and was on the plane in January. They wasted no time recruiting me.

"I came in '75, just after the flower children, and I grew up in London with fashion. I went for my interview there wearing a cute little dress and heeled shoes. The recruiter looked me up and down and said, 'Do you know where you're going? You're going to Newfoundland.' I said I knew where I was going and told her about the two physicians who showed us photos and did a good orientation. She said, 'We'll send you to St. Anthony. You might get a hair dresser there even if you don't get your fashion clothes.' I went to North West River and then Nain, so I was as far from fashion or a hair dresser as you could go. But that didn't matter.

"I flew to Goose Bay and the airport seemed no bigger than a shed. A medical student on the plane had been to Goose Bay and told me it was about three-quarters of an hour to get to North West River. I got paged over the intercom and went to the desk. This guy who seemed really huge was there. He didn't introduce himself, just said, 'Where are your bags?' My bags were really heavy, but he picked them up like they were feathers and started to walk. I trotted behind him thinking, 'You don't have a clue who this fellow is or where he's going.' I was scared but still followed him. I decided to ask him how long it took to get to North West River and if he didn't say three-quarters of an hour I'd know something wasn't right. We walked across the tarmac and I caught up and said, 'How long will it take to get to North West River?' He said, 'Fifteen minutes!' I thought, 'There's something very wrong!' I asked how we were getting there, and he pointed to a little red kite sitting on the runway. It was a little Beaver plane. I never saw anything so small! He threw my bags in the back and told me to get in front. As I'm sitting there it felt like the plane was going up one side and over the top of me. We took off and he's pumping by his side. I'm thinking, 'My God, he has to pump to keep the plane up.' Then he said, 'Would you pump this up and down?' By now I'm thinking, 'If I don't pump this right we're going to go down!' We were pumping up the wheels because we were landing on skis. As we came into North West River all I saw was a frozen river, something we don't have in England. I'm thinking, 'We're going to crash and go through the ice.' But we skied along nicely and stopped. By now I'm asking, 'What have I got myself into?' A guy came up alongside of the plane on a machine with a box behind it. It was a Ski-Doo, but I'd never seen a Ski-Doo in my life. He welcomed me and said, 'Jump on the machine.' I'm wondering, 'Do I sit forward or backwards?' I decided to wait until he got on to get some direction. Then he said, 'Climb on and hang onto me.'

"He took me to Shoush House, which was the hospital residence where five of us lived. There were two nursing assistants, and God bless their socks, they were really sweet and so welcoming. They said, 'Go and unpack and we'll make a cup of tea.' I came back and they start talking. I'm thinking, 'I came to Canada because they speak English, but I don't have a clue what they're saying.' They were speaking like we do but it was the accent and they spoke so fast. I sat there for the whole cup of tea nodding and shaking my head.

"The hospital was divided into two areas: pediatrics and a general area which included obstetrics. If you were on the general side you were responsible for emergencies that came in. On pediatrics there was one nurse during the day and at night the nurse was responsible for all areas. The people were wonderful to work with and I adapted quickly to the dialect, although I had problems with some of the sayings. The time sheet said, 'lunch at ten o'clock,' which I thought was early. Eventually I asked the head nurse, 'If I have lunch at ten o'clock and don't get off until eight this evening, I'm going to be starved. How come lunch is so early?' She was English and chuckled, then said, 'Lunch is your morning coffee or afternoon tea.'

"I was responsible for deliveries but couldn't suture, whereas at home I did suturing and episiotomies. After one delivery the lady needed stitching, so I said to the nursing assistants, 'I'm going to knock up the doctor.' They went into stitches laughing, so I asked why. Of course they were laughing because of what it means here versus what it meant to me. It was a really interesting time.

"We walked to the hospital through a wooded path. I was scared walking down there, which was silly because it was safer than anywhere else in the world. But I'd always think, 'You'd never walk a wooded street alone at home.' Then one night I saw the northern lights and thought I had died and gone to heaven. It was the most beautiful sight I ever saw in my life!

"North West River was the local hospital then, not Goose Bay, so we did escorts. We flew from there to pick up patients. I went to Cartwright to pick up a patient on a stretcher. I was so excited! As a little girl we listened to a program from Australia called *Flying Doctor*! I couldn't believe I was seeing this way of nursing. The nurse brought the patient down on a komatik and I was amazed. It was my first escort so the patient was stable. I enjoyed every minute because it really brought out your nursing and personal skills.

"Grenfell increased the nurses to three in Nain and was looking for someone to go. I volunteered because I thought it would be an interesting experience. Little did I know I'd be there eight years! I went for three weeks at first because they were giving three nurses a try. The head nurse was Irish and there was another English nurse. There wasn't a bedroom for a third nurse, so I slept in a three-bed guest room until the workmen arrived. Then they got that room and I slept in a three-bed men's ward.

"Working in Nain was totally different from North West River. We were more independent. But I was very independent anyway, because in my teaching hospital we relied on doctors as a lead. But midwives were expected to be independent of the doctors. In Nain we were supported by the doctors, but they wanted nurses to be independent and only use them on an on-call basis. It was nice working there.

"I was immensely homesick the first four months, but I enjoyed my work and loved working with different people. We worked like general practitioners and three of us were on-call all day. We got one day off a week and did one shift where we came Friday night and didn't get off until Sunday morning. We also did a split shift, and in the beginning the head nurse took that shift until I got used to things. We had clinic in the morning and she was always available. I did afternoon clinic alone but she was upstairs. I was exhausted running up and down-stairs asking questions but she was so patient. We shared the downstairs clinic with the dentist and put a screen on wheels across the middle. He worked on one side and we worked on the other. We didn't have a translator, so if we needed something translated we got somebody from the waiting room because they all spoke Inuktitut. This was someone from the community, so the gossip was something. Talk about patient confidentiality! Also the dental patients heard everything I discussed with my patients. They all said 'nakurmiik' and I asked the dentist what it meant, but he didn't know. I asked one of the aides who looked at me like, 'Are you for real?' It was 'thank you.' I got used to the language and could understand everything the clients said but couldn't speak to them.

"Clinics were a mish-mash of everything. We had four aides who worked upstairs with patients we kept in hospital and prayed the plane would get in or the weather would be good enough to get them out. To this day if I hear a helicopter in the sky, I have a huge feeling of relief! A lot of the children had otitis media [ear infections] and the biggest thing we did was check ears. I'd never done that before so learning it was a challenge. All we did was clean them, give antibiotics, and send them to St. Anthony. We had as high as 12 children go for grommets at a time. I think how sad that was because we put them on the plane without their moms and dads. They wore a big label saying who they were, and we hoped they wouldn't pass their coats around. They'd be gone two and three weeks where they couldn't fly back because of pressure with the tubes. That was a horrible thing!

"Parents in Nain didn't know how to look after their children at home when they got sick. As soon as a child got a fever they were brought to the hospital. They didn't know how to use Tylenol, cough syrup, aspirin, or anything, so we really needed a public health nurse. I went back to North West River for a couple of weeks before going to Nain permanently. A public health nurse came with me. One of the first things she did was teach the parents about caring for their children and we really pushed it in clinic.

"When my contract was up I went home to England to decide what I'd do. I had no intention of staying but the people were fantastic to work with and by then I'd met somebody. Within a month I decided I wanted to come back. Unfortunately the marriage ended, but fortunately I have a gorgeous daughter. I found the Inuit were very warm and caring. They took us into their hearts and involved us in anything they could. One of their big things was celebrating a 50th birthday. I went to one and couldn't understand why it was so sad and depressing. I asked an aide, because you got information about the culture from them. She said if you reached 50 and were well, there was a huge celebration, but if you reached 50 and were sick, then they had a wake with you there. I don't know if that still happens, but back in '75 it's what they did. Everybody in the community was invited, which was about 800 to 1,000 people. There was an order for people to go in and a time for them to turn up. They'd start off with people like the nurses because we were special in the community. I didn't see myself as special but they did. The nurses were one of the best guests, so they got the best china and the first of the food. Also a little shot of something that tasted like raw alcohol, although I never knew what it was. I always managed to leave it because I didn't want to get involved with it.

"Most of the nurses only stayed a year because Grenfell paid their fare out. So when I became head nurse, I knew we needed more nurses so staff wouldn't leave. We increased to six nurses and every nurse got one week off a month. Then they could leave the community, because Nain was quite stressful. We were often involved in incidents resulting from abuse and violence like stitching up somebody after a fight or alcohol abuse. Sexually transmitted diseases was another challenge because I'd never come into contact with it in practice.

"I got a call from a friend that there'd been a fight and somebody was dead on the floor. It was about three in the morning and the aide said, 'You can't go to that part of town by yourself.' I phoned the Mountie who said, 'He's drunk and doesn't know what he's talking about. Buddy is just passed out. Go back to bed.' The young fellow called back and said the same thing, so I phoned the Mountie again. He still didn't believe me, so I said, 'I know he's right. I'm taking my bag and going,' and hung up. The aide kept saying, 'You can't go by yourself,' but I'm thinking, 'They won't do anything to the nurse because this is their future health.' With that, there was a scuffle in the porch, which was the Mountie, who ran to the nursing station because he wasn't having me go alone. The guy had been murdered! That was my first time being involved in that kind of situation. It went to court and we had to say what we saw. In most cases the Mounties brought in a special investigation team and coached us on how to write up a statement. They were excellent and so supportive of us. The Mounties, social workers, and nurses in Nain worked really well together. We'd be subpoenaed to go to Goose Bay, so we had to get relief while we were in court. We would sit two or three days and not get called. That wasn't the best experience.

"We only had a radio and a telephone. The phone came on at nine in the morning and went off at nine at night. We used the RT to phone North West River, and every morning we'd get on that, but so did everybody else in the community. We learned a code to talk to the doctor about a client then he'd phone back and tell you what to do. It was really hard hiding who or what you were dealing with.

"We had a patient who'd been hit in the eye with a hockey puck. We were worried about hemorrhage and called the doctor. It was 9:00 p.m. when we finished so the phone shut down. He'd said to lay the patient flat, which didn't seem right, so we looked it up in the

Merck Manual and sat him up. I had my midwifery book and a *Merck Manual* for reference. That was it! I worshiped that *Merck Manual*. It was like my Bible. I could tell you everything in it by the time I finished. Dead on nine o'clock the next morning, the phone rang and the doctor said, 'I know I said to lay him flat but tell me you didn't.' We said, 'No, we sat him up, you're fine.'

"When there was a movie in the town hall, one of the nurses would get a health education film and put them on at the start of a movie and in the interval. When they changed reels this nurse would run in and put on another film. One Sunday afternoon we got a call saying a young fellow was going around on a Ski-Doo shooting anything he could, like cats and dogs. The film *Billy the Kid* had been shown the night before! The next thing they come through the door with a young Inuit man who'd been shot through his arm with a 22. It missed every bone in his arm! It was clean and hardly bleeding so we took care of it. Then the Mounties arrived carrying a guy by all fours with his knee smashed with a bullet. He tried to shoot a Mountie, so the special constable shot him with a hunting rifle and the bullet exploded! It was three in the afternoon! Nain didn't have a runway so it was pushing it to get a plane from North West River and back there before dark. I remember thinking, 'Where do I start suturing?' Because there was nothing to suture and it was bleeding like anything! We put a tourniquet on and all I could do was pack it. He was royally drunk and we didn't dare give him medication. I didn't know if we were going to keep him alive. We called in the other nurse and she was on the phone with the doctor relaying to me what I should do. We tried to put IVs in his arm and leg to get fluid into him because we didn't have blood or pack cells. In the meantime the RCMP tried to keep him from jumping all over the place. Luckily the RCMP plane was only 20 minutes away so it came back and a nurse flew out with him.

"We had to order supplies which I'd never done in my life. We put in an annual order for medicines, bandages, food, and anything needed to survive in a nursing station, and got supplies twice a year. We couldn't find any record from the previous year so the other nurse and I did the order together. We checked how many bandages we used in a week and multiplied by 52. That was the only way to do it. I ordered dry goods for the clinic and a doctor sent back saying I'd over-estimated by 10 bandages! I'm thinking, 'How do you over-estimate when you don't know how many to get in the first place?' Antibiotics for the children came by plane, but one doctor was only interested in keeping within budget and would send just six bottles of an antibiotic. That was six individual doses for a two-week period, but we saw more than six kids needing antibiotics so we taught the parents how to take antibiotics apart and mix them in jam for the babies. That was the frugal side of IGA and it was a very difficult circumstance to work in!

"The supplies would arrive suddenly. Everything came by boat at the one time. They were delivered in a big truck and put at the end of the yard. Imagine grocery supplies for one year! We had to store them in the basement and put away the medications. Then the Mounties regularly checked the control drugs.

"Each spring a stream came down the hill, through the front door, through the basement, and out through the clinic. And every spring we dug a ditch to redirect the water around the nursing station. After four years we got a better system because I wasn't doing that every year. But when we did those things we gained the respect of the Inuit because they saw we were willing to work hard.

"When I came we probably had six inpatients all the time, but after eight years we had maybe two or so. We had influxes like when we had an outbreak of whooping cough where we had 30 children, three to an adult mattress, on the floor. To relieve us they sent in three helicopters and took some children out. Grenfell [IGA] weren't happy because they were bringing infected children into a hospital setting. But we had a week of it and everyone was absolutely exhausted.

"I learned the importance of religion from a patient's point of view in Nain, and it has influenced my life ever since. A young lass prematurely delivered her baby. In that situation, midwives traditionally do a quick blessing over them. It was something well-recognized in England. Some people in Nain were Moravian, which is a German religion similar to the United Church. The baby and mom were transferred to St. John's, but she lost the baby. What was worse was that the Moravian minister hadn't blessed the child, so it couldn't be buried in the graveyard in Nain. She had to bury her baby in St. John's and come back to Nain never able to visit her baby's grave. I quickly realized how the Moravian Church had woven its way through the traditions of the community and how important it was. After that if we had a serious situation I was quick to ask the parents if they wanted the minister to say a prayer.

"We had a boy of about eight or nine years come in having bad seizures and we couldn't stop them. We called North West River and gave him medications nurses didn't normally give. We kept giving the medications but weren't getting anywhere, and we didn't know why he was seizuring. There was no family history, he had never seizured before, and there was no smell of anything on him. We didn't know what else to do! I said to his mother, 'I'm not sure we're going to get him out of this. Would you like the minister to come?' He came and said a prayer over the child. I don't know if 30 minutes was enough time for the medication to work, but the seizures stopped and he didn't seizure afterwards. We discovered later he was sniffing gasoline, so the toxic fumes probably lessened in 30 minutes.

"We could deliver second to fifth babies, but the first and over five had to go to North West River. We had an Indian lady, married to a local fellow, in labour with her second baby. The delivery went perfectly with a beautiful baby boy, and the dad was bouncing around. Ten o'clock that night we still hadn't delivered the placenta, and we couldn't get her out to hospital. We could either do a manual removal with no anesthetic, and nobody had done that, or leave it and hope she didn't bleed too much. The phones were down so we couldn't call North West River. She went unconscious and we put in two IVs to give her fluid because we didn't have anything else. By 1:00 a.m. she was stable and not bleeding much but still unconscious. At the time I took in boarders, remembered one of them was a chopper pilot and had a radio. He called a mayday and someone in Halifax heard it and called Goose Bay. They switched on the RT because someone had accidentally switched it off.

"We kept her that night and the chopper took her out in the morning. It took a special stretcher which we didn't have, so the janitors decided to take a door off and put her on the door. I told the janitors to be careful because it wasn't a solid door. We brought her to the chopper in a van, then they had to take the chopper door off to get her in. The stretcher door was too wide to put the chopper door back on so they chopped out a piece. The nurse sat behind the pilot with the patient and a huge old-fashioned oxygen cylinder. The most she could do was look at the patient, feel her pulse, and have the pilot land if she had problems. They landed twice for more oxygen and to fix the IVs. I told North West River to put her on a regular stretcher. They didn't and the patient wakes up on the ice on North West River! They took her off the chopper on the door stretcher and it collapsed in the middle! Fortunately the woman survived! We kept the baby in Nain because there wasn't room in the chopper.

"You prayed the whole way out because you never knew what was going to happen. A few times we lost patients on the way out, which was very difficult. The chopper normally came from North West River. It was big and equipped and we could lay a stretcher in the back. We rarely got a chopper though because it was so expensive, but there were no roads so it was a plane or nothing.

"One of my responsibilities was taking x-rays. The Irish head nurse taught me how to take them, how to develop them with the old dip-in mechanism and how to read them. People were excited when we started because before, when someone had a suspected broken limb, they were sent out for x-rays only to discover they didn't have one. We also had fantastic doctors visit every month from North West River. We kept a list of patients to be referred if we didn't know what to do. They spent hours teaching us. They showed us things on x-rays so we knew what we were seeing. We did dental care because we had no dentist. He came every two months and taught us how to inject lidocaine into the gum or into back of the mouth and how to pull or temporarily fill a tooth until the patient went to North West River. I hated dental! I'd give the injection then walk around the nursing station because I was so nervous about pulling a tooth. I pulled a lot of teeth but it was not my favourite thing to do. I'd pray it wouldn't break because then the patient had to go out and dental cases were the lowest of the low to get on the plane. The plane had 10 seats and went to Nain, Davis Inlet, Hopedale, Makkovik, Rigolet, and Postville to pick up patients. There wasn't much chance you'd get on and everybody complained that Nain took all the seats.

"We were also taught to put in IUDs and to check eye pressure for glaucoma. I became very good at putting IVs and butterflies in the skull for infants and babies. We'd do assessments, trying to communicate with somebody in a different language, so when I became head nurse I got translators for the clinic. They were fantastic. I did public health in Nain for a while and repeatedly went back to one house, where there was scabies, doing teaching and leaving pamphlets. I didn't think anything about it until one day I said to an aide, 'This doesn't make sense because we're doing everything.' She said, 'You're leaving the English pamphlets and they don't speak English.' This girl took the main public health leaflets we used and translated them into Inuktitut. She did nursing and is now head nurse in Nain. I'm thrilled because it is so important they have one of their own who speaks fluently.

"In Public Health, I did a lice check every morning in a different school grade and treated them. It was a lot of work but worthwhile. Health teaching in the school took up most of our time because the only way to improve the health of Nain was through health education of the children. We also visited moms with new babies and the elderly to check blood pressure. These were more social assessments to see how they were doing. We were kept busy. We also got involved in other things like when government said the Inuit could only kill so many caribou a year. The Inuit by tradition are very frugal about how they catch caribou, much better than we are, and have a huge respect for preserving traditional animals. One person might kill six caribou but then share them between families of maybe 10. You couldn't buy fresh meat in Nain. It came in September and before long was freezer burned. The public health nurse for the Labrador Inuit Association asked me to write a statement why the caribou licensing was wrong. I wrote it and thought no more about it.

"An Assistant Deputy Minister came to Nain in January or February to check out the situation. Nain had three stores: a hardware store, a general convenience store which sold fresh meat in September and October, and the government store which had a freezer. We talked and I told him the truth about everything and his look says he thinks I'm nuts. I suggested he walk around the government store. He came back and said with a straight face, 'Do you realize the only thing fresh in this store is an onion?' They started to send fruits and vegetables, like eggplant, on a large plane which landed on the ice. The problem was that the native folks had never seen most of them before. All they knew was turnip, carrot, onion, potato, and cabbage. People bought the broccoli and cauliflower because, if it was being sold, it had to be good. Then we got lots of calls asking what to do with the vegetables. The caribou licensing thing was on CBC, but I hadn't gotten permission to make a statement. I got a call from my boss in St. Anthony! Fortunately he was a wonderful person and only tormented me about how shocked he was to hear the public health nurse in Nain had made a statement. I didn't know I made a statement because we didn't have TV.

"We had problems with the children in the summer because their mothers worked at the fish plant and the children were left to run around with no care. I started a daycare, which ran for one summer and it was very successful. We did a lot of health teaching and the people working there learned how to prepare a healthy meal. We tried to hand it over to the community the next year but it wasn't as successful. Then the following year there were the fishery problems so daycare wasn't needed. There was a lot of wife abuse and the community wanted a safe house. I went with them when they presented a paper to government on wife abuse and the need for a shelter.

"Nain didn't have running water or sewage, only slop banks out-side their homes. We tried a campaign, but I didn't know how to get the government in St. John's to see what life was like. I took photos of how close the slop banks were to the houses and the children playing around them and gave them to the council. I wrote a paper and included the pictures to present to government to get a cleanup. We never did get it! They built new houses and put in water and sewage, but they didn't get rid of the other ones. My daughter is very involved in Nain and she says most of those houses are gone now. But it's taken over 25 years to get there!

"After public health I went back to the hospital and we had a full-time doctor. It was very frustrating because she couldn't do blood tests and get results. We had a lady who was unconscious from a bad stroke and the doctor didn't know her electrolytes. Then she had another stroke and the doctor didn't know if she should resuscitate. We didn't have paddles to resuscitate or an EKG to see what her heart was doing! This doctor also thought we weren't doing enough about the violence in the community. My thinking was that we could support and encourage them, but it was important for the people to do it themselves and gradually they are. The Inuit move themselves forward very well.

"I went to St. Anthony in '81 to work in emergency. Suddenly I couldn't do things I had done in Nain, not even put on a band-aid by myself. It was an amazing change! All I did was shuffle patients in and out of rooms to see the doctor. I moved to Harbour Deep as public health nurse. There was no road but the most I had to get out was a broken leg. The people were the most wonderful people you'd ever want to nurse. From there I went to Roddickton as a Regional Nurse Supervisor, which was different again because there wasn't the violence—just the traditional stuff like heart disease.

"I had my first breech delivery in Roddickton. One morning I was the only midwife on and we had a lady in labour with her second baby. We didn't do deliveries but she was too close to go to St. Anthony. The doctor examined her and said the head was presenting well. But when I looked at the woman I thought, 'There's something not right,' and I was trying to think what I learned. The doctor had left to visit the outside communities so only myself and the other nurse were there. Fortunately, the two doctors I met at home before I came taught me things a midwife wouldn't normally do. I decided to do a vaginal exam even though I wasn't supposed to, because I knew I couldn't deliver the baby without knowing what's coming. I realized it wasn't the head but a bum! I knew I needed the mom's cooperation; if not, I didn't stand a chance. We didn't have forceps in the building! I told the other nurse to have oxygen ready the minute the baby came out. Afterwards she said she wondered why I said that, but when she saw my face and the terror in my eyes, she realized the presenting part was the bum and thought, 'We're not going to get a live baby.' I did a huge episiotomy and put my hands in as high as I could. I used my hands as a forceps to guide the head down and we had a delivery. The baby cried as soon as she came out, and the mother said, 'That was a different delivery from the last one.' This mom was fantastic!

"I got my degree at MUN and went back to St. Anthony to work for a year as nurse-in-charge of obstetrics where we did all the deliveries. Then I was in charge of Public Health for the region before I left to teach in Corner Brook.

"I've had the most amazing career anyone could wish for in Newfoundland and Labrador. I'm eternally grateful for the experiences I've had and wouldn't have gotten them if I'd stayed at home. I love the people I worked with and the client populations everywhere I've gone. It's a very different culture. I was lucky to be accepted into communities. I was only in Harbour Deep three months and they gave me a huge farewell shower when I left. I got so many presents I was embarrassed. It's been an experience with highs and lows and challenges you wouldn't believe, but it's been fantastic. Who would have known when I graduated that I'd land in Corner Brook teaching BN students? One sad thing is I've lost touch with my friends at home who have gone on with their own lives."

❋

Sue (nee Froude) Webb was born in Croydon, Surrey, England. She graduated from University College Hospital in London as a SRN in 1973. Following completion of midwifery as a SCM in Norwich, Norfolk, England, in 1974, she was recruited to work at North West River in 1975.

CATHIE (McFARLANE) LETHBRIDGE

✻

1975

*"It never occurred to me that flying around and being in charge at
27 or 28 was anything different. To me it was just daily occurrences and it
wasn't daunting. You did what you could and felt you were helping."*

"I wanted to go to Australia but my friend wanted to come to Canada.
We went to Australia House in London and it was pouring rain. We
chose the wrong tube stop and had to walk. By the time we got there
we were soaked. The man on the door said, 'We don't need nurses. We
need midwives. You can go upstairs.' By this time I was annoyed, which
wasn't his fault, but I thought, 'No I'm not!' So we came to Canada.

"There was an IGA advertisement in a London paper. It was totally
different from what we'd done before, so we decided to try it. We
wanted to come together to Goose Bay, but they had a small staff
and there weren't many positions. My friend came eight weeks after
me. We went to the Canadian Embassy, had an interview and a
medical. Everything was processed in eight weeks, which is nothing
compared to nowadays, and we got a work permit. I didn't know where
I was coming, but the day I arrived in Goose Bay was carnival day
and Frank Sinatra had just visited the base. The place was absolutely
hopping! I thought I was coming to a little secluded place and was

amazed with all that was going on!

"The maintenance man met me and took me to the hospital in their bus. The hospital was small but busy. It had about 20 beds, a nursery, two delivery rooms and a lot of pediatrics. A very tiny OR opened off the corridor and ICU was a cubby hole meant to store oxygen cylinders! We'd put the head of the bed into the corridor so we could see the patient from the nursing station. When I came to the old hospital we only did operations when it wasn't raining because water dripped through the lights onto the OR table.

"The day after I arrived I had to fly to Montreal on a commercial flight with a woman who had acute abdominal pain. The base surgeon was gone and there was no back-up surgeon. Halfway to Montreal she had acute diarrhea and vomiting! Here I was in a strange country, winging my way to a place I'd never been before, with a girl who didn't speak English! I brought her to the hospital and caught a plane back. I've done similar trips hundreds of times since.

"The nurses, visiting doctors and public health nurse lived upstairs in the residence while the doctors had houses behind that building. An older nurse who was extremely religious lived in residence and at Easter she made baskets with handmade cards and put them outside our doors in the corridor. One of the visiting doctors went to the communal bathroom in the middle of the night, put his foot in the Easter eggs and went down on the floor! We had lots of parties and dressed up. It was a good life for young girls because there was a lot of activity at the base. We worked hard and we played hard!

"We had four midwives, which weren't enough to cover the shifts, so we worked during the day and did call at night. We did eight-hour shifts and whoever worked evenings also covered nights. We slept during the day if we were up at night. Once we were up five nights in a row, which was five 16-hour shifts. There was no union then. I don't remember my salary but that wasn't important. I didn't bother as long as I had enough to live on. It was the adventure. We did everything. One minute you'd be in outpatients treating somebody with an overdose, and the next you might have a delivery, then leave to give meds on pediatrics. Everything was together so if you were the nurse, you were the nurse!

"I never understood why they brought nurses from England to be in charge. I was here about three months when the charge nurse left, and I got it because no one else wanted it. The few local nurses on staff worked part-time, took each summer off and came back to work for the winter. Being in charge included looking after the pharmacy, which I found a challenge, and organizing rotations. As I was doing all this I thought, 'I might as well get paid for it.' After four months I became Director of Nursing but still had to be on call. Then I was in charge of diets, organizing visiting specialists and their clinics along with the administrative stuff. Things were totally different in administration because my fingers were in all the pies. I was responsible for every department 24 hours a day.

"We had a man who needed special antibiotics which we didn't have, and I was on the phone night and day trying to get them. Making sure we had enough medication was stressful because it usually came from the government depository in St. John's. If it was out of the ordinary it might come from Montreal. There were three flights a week so you had to make sure there was enough medication. Vaccines were another thing we had to have because there was a lot of rabies along the coast. Fortunately we didn't see a lot of rabies, but we did see gas gangrene because people didn't take care of themselves. We also saw botulism from seal meat that hadn't been properly frozen.

"When I got here the plans for a new hospital extension had been drawn up. Then the Americans pulled out and offered us the base hospital. People were disappointed that government wouldn't build the new addition, but I was new and didn't know about that. I organized the move to the military hospital. I've done that twice since but the first time was interesting. The new hospital had 40 beds, a proper OR with an autoclave, and an ICU with piped-in oxygen for three beds. It was a great improvement. Also, the basement didn't flood with sewage, which was a vast improvement! But then we had cockroaches and silverfish, which we didn't before. The hospital was bigger and built in an H shape. It was spread out, so if we had an emergency, it was a long way between areas. We had five nurses in emergency/outpatients and about seven doctors who were salaried. They ran outpatient clinics during the day and covered emergency. It was tremendously busy, especially if we had an emergency or an accident.

"There were two units with midwives in one section because there were a lot of military families and a lot of deliveries. We had positions for seven midwives but only ever had five at most, so we also staffed it with nursing assistants or nurses. The military families would come in and turn up their nose about midwives, but we'd talk to them and they'd get interested. By the end of their experience they were saying, 'For my first baby I was in stirrups and it was horrible. This was so much nicer!' I enjoyed hearing that and never heard them say anything bad!

"In the nursing unit there were about 10 staff and two part-time nurses in the OR. The OR only ran until about 1:00 p.m., so they did night call. We also had five local nursing assistants. There were at least two nurses on days and one on evenings and nights. I spent a lot of time relieving for lunch or doing an odd night.

"When North West River hospital closed we started to do mede-vacs, and at first there was only RT operations to the coast. Emergency evacuations from the coast weren't common because the nurse tried to deal with it herself since she couldn't always get through on the RT and we were very dependent on weather. There was only one plane and it was very difficult to organize transport.

"Shortly before I arrived, a man came into the hospital and shot his wife dead in the bed, and people were still very traumatized by that. Then the RCMP would bring in people who we had to subdue. Some-body held them down and I gave the needle though their clothes. I was horrified by it! Looking back, there were a lot of women who I think were abused and being used by the military. They'd go berserk, which might have been because of a mental illness, but more likely it was abuse. It was very sad.

"We had a teenage boy whose parents were out of town and he was putting weed killer on the garden for them. He was siphoning it from a big can into a small one by sucking a pipe to start the flow and must have ingested some. We phoned St. John's to find out what to do because we didn't have poison control then. I think we gave him atropine and the doctor kept saying, 'This is going to kill him.' Evidently the stuff came out through the skin, so we kept washing him and giving him lethal doses of atropine although we knew the danger. Luckily the doctor saved him.

"In 1976 the hospital plane was charted by Hydro and crashed on the ice in North West River with six people on board. Only two survived. We sent staff over a gravel road to evacuate people, which was a big deal because we didn't have many to send. They went across the river by cable car because there was no bridge. One young girl who wasn't paralyzed when she reached North West River was by the time she got to Halifax. They had no choice but to get her off the ice.

"We had a young boy who slipped on the ice and must have injured himself internally. We opened outpatients and put a call on the radio for blood because we didn't have any blood transfusion services. We had to do all sorts of things, and I was with him well into the early hours. My job was to take blood from people and get as much as we could. We used 14 units that night, but unfortunately the boy died. It was vascular and we just couldn't do anything.

"I stayed in Labrador because I loved the work and it was never boring. Also I married and had two children, and after my husband left, I knew I could support my children here. I had a house and enjoyed my job and it's a nice place to bring up children. I retired in 2004 and spent that summer in my house in Harbour Grace. Then I came back here for the winter and loved it because I spent it skiing. After a year of retirement, I thought, 'What am I doing?' I went back to Harbour Grace but Goose Bay called and said, 'We're short of midwives, would you come back and give it a try?' I upgraded my clinical skills and am back doing midwifery and love it. I'm considered casual but work full-time.

"I go back to England frequently but not to stay because England has changed tremendously. I've worked here 40 years. It never occurred to me that flying around and being in charge at 27 or 28 was anything different. To me it was just daily occurrences and it wasn't daunting. You did what you could and felt you were helping. I've had a good career and it's certainly been very interesting and varied. I'm glad I was a nurse and loved every minute of it."

❀

Catherine (nee McFarlane) Lethbridge was born in London, England. She graduated as a SRN from the Royal Naval Hospital in Portsmouth, England, in 1968. In 1971, she completed midwifery as a SCM from the Southern General Hospital in Glasgow, Scotland, and completed a six-month neonatal course before immigrating to work at Goose Bay Hospital in 1975.

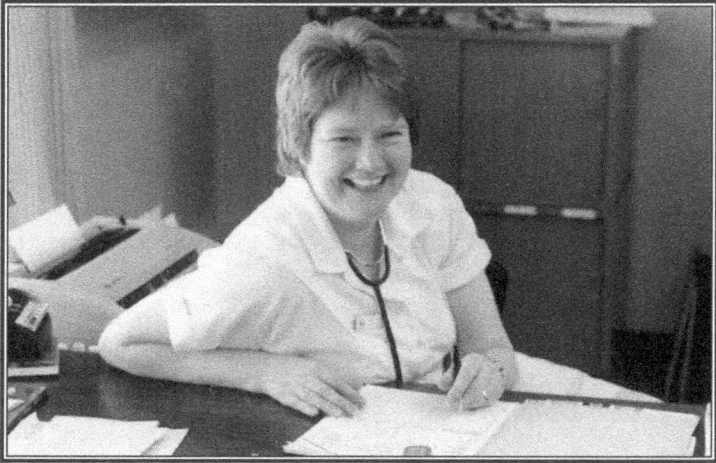

RUTH (TREES) SAMPSON

❋

1978

"I got a call to come to 236 quick. I thought, 'What is 236?'
It was a telephone number and I was supposed to know where it was!"

"I was in Zambia and my friend heard about the Grenfell mission, so four of us applied but only two came. I went home for three months before coming to Port Hope Simpson in October. My friend came later to go to Hopedale. She had Christmas with me then went north but didn't stay long.

"I was interviewed in an old house in London with a narrow winding stairway up to a lady's office. I asked what clothing I needed and stuff like that, but she didn't give me the details I needed. I got my parka from Eddie Bauer and other clothing when I got here.

"When I arrived in Gander, I thought, 'What have I come to!' The pilot of our DWT plane met me. It was a small executive, medevac plane which took me to St. Anthony. I had two weeks' orientation in St. Anthony, which didn't help, and I complained bitterly. The person doing the orientation said she didn't know what to give me because I had so much experience, which was absolute nonsense because I had no suitable experience for here. I had never done physical assessment or breath sounds because we weren't taught that in training, and they should have known I needed that. I had no idea what I needed, but I gave her a list of things like suturing. She took the list and ignored it! I spent three or four days with the dentist because we were supposed to remove teeth, but soon afterwards we weren't allowed to do it. I watched him fit people for dentures and do fillings but thought, 'I'm not going to need this.' I stopped going because it was a waste of my time. The orientation was useless and I couldn't believe nobody else complained. I felt so out of my depth and I didn't like the feeling because I wanted to be on top of everything.

"I flew to Port Hope Simpson on a Saturday in the Grenfell float plane because there was no ice. I had to clamber down to the dock, get on the float, then into the plane. We landed in every place on the way up and got to Port Hope Simpson about half past 11:00. We landed on water. I thought, 'Dear God. What have I come to?'

"I was the nurse-in-charge. Can you believe it? The nurse already there met the plane. She never offered me a cup of coffee and I hadn't had lunch. She went into all the stuff I needed to know because she was leaving on Monday, although she was to stay until Wednesday. It was ridiculous! She'd been there six weeks and was disgruntled because she wanted to stay but they appointed me. She plowed me with all of this information and we did one clinic together. I got on the RT, although I didn't know how to work the mike. I asked the doctor in St. Anthony, 'What do I do? Who gives RT the authority to change orientation plans? I've only had half a day clinic with her.' She stayed until Wednesday, but that's all the orientation I got. Then she took off!

"The phones weren't very good then so we had CB sets and called each station every morning. We discussed any problems, but we didn't discuss patients if possible because all the stations could hear. Sometimes we had no choice because the phones were out half the time. That was quite the eye opener!

"When I had my first patient I didn't know where to find the drugs. I didn't even know the names of drugs because they were different. In orientation I asked about giving hemleaf for a fracture and the doctor said 282s would be all right. I didn't know what 282s were but I decided not to show my ignorance and find out later. My biggest challenges were the names of medication and physical assessment because I didn't have a clue! I'd never diagnosed before, but I had enough sense to know I was out of my depth. I expressed my concerns and prayed a lot.

"Port Hope Simpson is north of St. Anthony. People from Britain came here for the wood and when they pulled out; people fished here in the summer. When I came, there were about 600 people and it was completely cut off. The only transportation was by air.

"It was a one-nurse station. A nurse from the community relieved every Thursday so I had Thursdays off. She also did call one night from home and one weekend. I did the other three. It was horrendous because it seemed I was always on call. I should have had her help for a couple of weeks but I didn't utilize her properly. I just plowed on!

"One of my first emergencies was a lady with pre-eclampsia. She was in clinic overnight and flown out the next day. I handled that okay because of my midwifery skills. Prior to opening the clinic, the nearest one was Mary's Harbour. The doctors came every six weeks and I held some patients until they came. Diabetic refills and BP checks was why most people came to the clinic. I wondered if anybody had a band-aid because people came with minor wounds! I saw an enormous number of patients for trivia. The people in Port Hope Simpson had been self-sufficient until they got the clinic; then became very dependent on it. My friend and I presented a paper on that at a Circumpolar Health Conference in Copenhagen.

"One night when the plane came, we went to see the pilot even though the waiting room was full. That was the highlight of the day! He brought the mail to all the communities so we always went to say hi and get the news. One day shortly after I came he said, 'Hop in!' and took me to Norman Bay where I met the nurse. She was Scottish and we became friends. Norman Bay was a very poor community with 47 people. She came down the hill with two Labrador suitcases, which are black garbage bags, and got on the plane. She was relieving in Charlottetown and was planning to do her laundry there. We flew her to Charlottetown and then back to Port Hope Simpson. It took less than an hour, but things like that were a light relief.

"I had a four-month-old baby die. Her mother was the lady with pre-eclampsia. That was the most horrendous experience because I didn't have a clue what was wrong with her. She died from an overwhelming viral pneumonia. I never felt so helpless in my life! I'd only been here four months and thought if I had more experience I might have sent her out earlier, but I don't know if she would have survived. We couldn't fly the baby out because of weather ... I was determined to send her for autopsy, but the parents only wanted to bury her. I pleaded with them to send her out. It was dreadful! We got a new TV and the box was in the garage. We packed the baby in snow in this box. It was so stormy that the other RN, who was on call, got lost going to a patient's house. I don't think she worked after that, but the experience had a horrible effect on both of us. When the pilot arrived he apologized that he couldn't get in, and I burst into tears. He went back and told the supervisor to see to me. I resigned because I couldn't handle it. I wrote a letter and said I was totally ill equipped. My dad was visiting and I told them I was going home with him. I agreed to come for a year and I don't recall signing a contract. Apparently it was a gentleman's agreement and not binding. I got a nice letter from one of the doctors telling me about times when he felt inadequate. Then someone from nursing called and said they didn't want to accept my resignation. They gave me a week's holiday before Dad left and a week's orientation in Flower's Cove.

"I went to Flower's Cove and realized I was probably doing as well as any of the nurses. By the time I got there I knew what I needed to learn. I did a lot of medevacs there because whenever the ambulance went to St. Anthony they wanted to send me, but I told them I was there to work with the doctor, although I did go with midwifery cases. I had to put my foot down sometimes!

"I had a call from the nurse in Norman's Bay wanting me to call St. Anthony because she had an emergency in Charlottetown and couldn't get through. The ice wasn't good enough to go by Ski-Doo so she needed the plane to take her while there was still enough light. I called St. Anthony and they told me to go because we could get there by Ski-Doo. Four of us went, including the dentist and the public health nurse. It was a lengthy trip and took forever! When we arrived, the man's foot had coats around it. When we took off the dressing, blood was squirting, so obviously an artery had gone. We replaced the dressing and the dentist and I got an IV in. The cut was a half inch but we couldn't find the bleeding point. The dentist extended the wound, found the artery and tied it off. Talk about the Lord giving me help when I needed it! If he hadn't been there, I would have had to keep deep pressure on it and fly him out the next day. I decided to go back that night before I got too stiff to get on the Ski-Doo. We left about two in the morning and it was really cold. The public health nurse got her feet frozen so we stopped at a cabin. My future husband and one of his friends came to meet us and they lit a fire. We got her feet warmed up and went on. We got back about four in the morning but my husband's friend wasn't with us. He ran out of gas and they had to go look for him! I had them call me when they got back. It was all very exciting!

"I had no problem understanding the people in Port Hope Simpson, but it was a community of white settlers. There were no natives although people do have native blood. I had a lady in the clinic and when I asked what was wrong, she said, 'I've got a wonderful pain in my pole.' I worked in Africa and didn't know the language, but patients pointed to where the pain was—but this woman gave no indication. I excused myself and asked one of the receptionists, 'What's your pole?' She pointed to the back of her head. I went back and said, 'Tell me about your headache.' People spoke English but so fast! At coffee I didn't have a clue what people were saying. My brother-in-law was the maintenance man and he drove me everywhere because I didn't know where places were. He mumbled and I couldn't understand him. I'd say, 'Pardon?' and he'd repeat it, but I was too embarrassed to say pardon more than twice. He mocked my British accent but I'd say, 'If you didn't mumble I'd be able to understand you.' So I did have difficulty in that sense. Another time I got a call to come to '236' quick. I thought, 'What is 236?' It was a telephone number and I was supposed to know where it was!

"The clinic truck in Port Hope Simpson was a big Ford Suburban. The maintenance man left it at the clinic for me the weekend after I arrived but I hadn't driven it. On Friday evening I got a call from a lady saying, 'Nurse, you've got to come, Suzy's sick.' I asked what she meant but she kept saying, 'She's sick, Nurse. Come!' She was having a baby! They would say so-and-so is due to be sick on a certain day, which was the delivery date. I asked where she lived because I had to drive, and it was near a house I knew so I told her to wait on the road. I picked her up and when we got to the boyfriend's house the girl was upstairs. Meanwhile the mother and boyfriend were like red rags to a bull. He went berserk! As soon as I saw the girl, I knew she wasn't in labour but I wanted to check her. I don't think the boyfriend intended to, but he hit me in the head and I literally saw stars. It was all over the community in no time that he hit the new nurse! We had to get the girl home but he didn't want her to go. One of the men saw the clinic truck and came in. He drove the girl, her mother, and me to their home where I did a proper examination. The man drove me back to our truck and jokingly said, 'Stay on the right.' It was a narrow dirt road so you could only drive down the middle. I tried to stay on the right but went off the road and the front tire ended up in a stream. I walked to the clinic to phone someone to help, and my [future] husband and his friend came to help. That's how I met him—as a damsel in distress! It wasn't love at first sight but we had lots of fun.

"Shortly after I came to Port Hope Simpson I did a clinic in Williams Harbour, which was a year-round satellite community of Port Hope Simpson. We took a box for medicines and charts, and one of the part-time girls helped to get everything together. The maintenance man, the public health nurse, and I went in a speedboat, and I'd never been in a boat that size. There was a swell on the water and we had to clamber up over the rocks in William's Harbour. We did clinic in a house owned by the community's lay dispenser. Somebody went through the community to tell people the nurse was here. It was impossible to do a proper clinic and I was never good at it, although I did get more organized. We never knew how long to wait for people so I'd go to the houses to see if anybody was sick. We'd leave at 7:00 a.m. and wouldn't get back until midnight. The maintenance man got overtime and I didn't, but that changed and we both got it in the end.

"The women came back from the summer satellite communities to Port Hope Simpson each winter so the kids could go to school. But because William's Harbour was a year-round community, we did clinics there every six weeks in the winter. But that was a waste of time because I'd bring the box of tricks, charts, and medicines, and people would come on weekends for drug refills! I had to work on the weekend and we didn't get call-back pay then. They weren't supposed to do that, but they did. It was unbelievable!

"When my husband and I were going out together, I did a stint in

Hopedale and some relief in Mary's Harbour and in Charlottetown. He did maintenance relief for three summers, a month each in Port Hope Simpson, Charlottetown, and in Black Tickle. When he was in Charlottetown I'd swap with the nurse there and she'd come here. We did that on our own and told St. Anthony afterwards.

"I also did a stint in Davis Inlet, which was absolutely dreadful. I was going on vacation with a friend, but she didn't have the right visa so we couldn't go. My relief had already replaced me and I didn't want to take three weeks work from her, so I relieved a nurse in Davis Inlet. The place was horrendous! When I arrived the sewer had backed up into the basement, and she was on the RT screaming, 'There's S-H-I-T in the basement,' only she wasn't spelling it out. The plumber came on the plane and they sent out a canoe to get him. He wouldn't get off the plane because the water was too rough so he went back. She was so frustrated! I got my first mosquito bites there, and my feet and face were swollen and unrecognizable. The RCMP had a house and we'd shower there because the water in the station was awful. You couldn't even stay in the toilet very long it was so bad. It was dreadful! Then the other nurse got sick and I was exhausted because patients came to the clinic all hours of the day and night. A lady with a bandage on her nose came at 9:00 p.m. for a dressing. I told her the clinic times and sent her away. She came back with her husband who said, 'You don't understand; she's come for a dressing.' I said, 'I'm sorry. The clinic is closed. Come back.' He wasn't pleased but he left. Every IV fluid there was out-of-date. They medevaced the nurse out and I was left by myself. It was summer and people, like the nuns and teachers that the nurses usually associated with, were gone.

"My husband is from Port Hope Simpson and has nine siblings. We were married here from the clinic. My mom was 80-something so she couldn't come, and my husband would have been out of his depth getting married in England. We lost three babies but we had one boy with Down's syndrome. He's 22 now and absolutely fantastic. The first year we were married we lived in St. Anthony because I had a joint appointment with MUN and he went back to school. We stayed in St. Anthony two years. I liked it because we were back and forth all the time, but my husband didn't.

"I wanted the maintenance man to make me a coach box because if the plane brought freight when he was gone, we had to go to the plane with a komatik. I couldn't tie stuff on the komatik, so I wanted a coach box where I could put stuff. But he wouldn't make one. One night his brother and sister were badly burned in a little house where they played. He was 12 and she was two. The boy got out with burns on his face and hands, but the girl had really deep burns. I usually finished clinic about 7:00 p.m. and had just sat down to eat when the doorbell rang. When I opened the door, the girl was there with the skin off her face and hands. We couldn't fly them out because it was foggy, so we were up all night doing dressings and whatever. I phoned St. Anthony to get the IV and medication regime to make them comfortable because the boy was in pain where his burns were super-ficial. The pilot was stuck in Mary's Harbour so I phoned him, told him what happened, and said not to go back without coming here. The next thing, I woke up to his voice. Because he could see the oil tanks, he'd flown that night in the fog because he wanted to fly out as soon as he could. The next morning both kids had terrible edema. I was scared because she had edema around her throat. About 6:00 a.m. the pilot decided to go. Meanwhile I said to the maintenance man, 'Now we might get a coach box,' and in two days I had a beautiful one. Both kids survived, but that was an awful night!

"I decided to do the nurse practitioner program. When I came back the only nurse-in-charge positions were at Port Hope Simpson, Nain, or Hopedale, but I said no. I wanted Forteau because I knew the place and I liked it, but Grenfell didn't want me to go. I went back to Port Hope Simpson. First when we lived there, my husband was fishing. He came home on weekends, but I was usually working or on call so it wasn't good for family life. He still fished in the summer, so it was the same when we went back this time except I lost a baby at 20 weeks. The nursing supervisor visited me in hospital and I said, 'The next vacancy in Forteau is mine and I'm going to pull seniority.' I got the next position! We moved there for family life and my husband fished from Forteau. We built a house there but then the moratorium came.

"I've practiced nursing in Newfoundland for 24 years. I can't believe I stayed as long as I did. I was happy I was a nurse. I was 23 when I started. My mom died in '88, and afterwards I didn't go home because she had died, my sister had moved, and I sold my house there. For the first time I felt I was going to be a visitor in my home country. I didn't go back for 16 years. Then in 2004 we had my 40-year nursing reunion, which was my motivation to go back. The family went and we had a great holiday. It was good.

"I'm glad I came to Newfoundland. Everything has worked out really well. We bought an RV and have land in Forteau so we go there each summer. We have the best of both worlds. I'm content in Port Hope Simpson, but when I go out I always think, 'How will I cope with being back there?' Winter here is horrendous!"

❃

Ruth (nee Trees) Sampson was born in Darlington, England. She graduated as a SRN from Guy's Hospital in London in 1967. In 1969, she completed midwifery as a SCM from St. James Hospital in Leeds, England. Before immigrating to work at the Port Hope Simpson nursing station in 1977, she completed a one-year Public Health (Health Visiting) course at Leeds University.

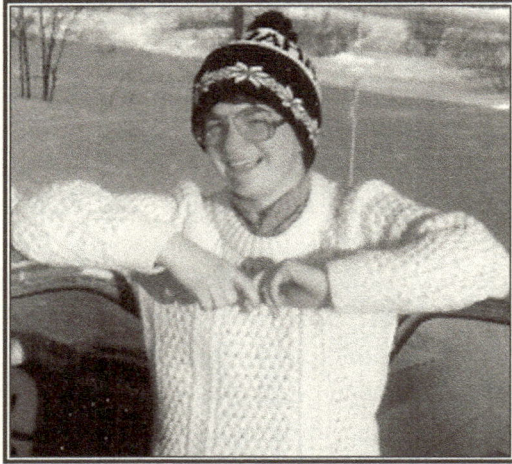

MAGGIE (ARKELL) LINSTEAD

❀

1981

*"We lived and worked in the old nursing station,
so it was 24/7! You even worked on your 'so-called' day off
if it got busy. We were never away from work!"*

"I wanted to travel after I finished midwifery. I worked about six months to get as much delivery experience as possible because I wanted to work in a 'wild and wooly place.' I wanted to go to a rural area for adventure because I lived in London and knew what a big city was like. I looked at New Zealand, Australia, and South Africa but not Canada. During midwifery I contacted a friend who worked with Grenfell in Labrador and was home to visit. She told me about working in the nursing stations and it sounded so exciting and different. I thought,

'That's what I'm going to do.' She had pictures of the winter pastimes like Ski-Dooing, ice fishing, and flying around in the single-engine planes.

"When my friend returned to Labrador she told her supervisor that a newly qualified midwife was interested in coming. They were desperate for nurses on the coast so it wasn't long before they contacted me. It was about 12 months from the time I saw my friend until I came here. Grenfell really got things moving!

"I landed in Gander in September and it was so windy the plane couldn't fly from St. Anthony to get me. I thought that was strange because it was beautiful sunny weather in Gander. I went by bus to Deer Lake and from there to St. Anthony on a bus called the 'Viking Express.' It was anything but an express! I was spared the rough spots because the bus driver told me, 'You'll get a good ride because it's paved all the way now.' I arrived in St. Anthony at midnight, absolutely beat but very excited.

"I spent two weeks there getting an orientation to the hospital and being introduced to the nursing and medical staff I would be communicating with when I went to Labrador. I did assessments in outpatients because I hadn't worked as a community nurse or done out-post nursing and they reviewed things like suturing. One anesthetist said, 'You're a midwife so you need to know how to do a pudendal block.' I remember thinking, 'I don't think I'll be doing those.' But he showed me how to do it while I'm praying I'd never have to do one. And I didn't!

"I was introduced to Newfoundland culture in my first two weeks but not to the language. When I went to Forteau I found a big difference between people in St. Anthony and people in Labrador. It wasn't until I went there that I felt I met the real people. St. Anthony is unique because it's full of people who came from somewhere else. Only a small proportion has lived there all their lives and many of them went to the Grenfell school. Also they had a lot of contact with the people who worked in the hospital.

"Nursing in St. Anthony was familiar because many of the nurses came from Britain, although medications had different names. The two nurses in Forteau were also British, which softened the blow a bit. My main difficulty was understanding people when they came to clinic. They spoke very fast and ran their words together. I couldn't understand what they said! I thought they spoke like people from Devon in the west country of England, and that's where many of their ancestors came from. Almost everybody was related, so you had to be careful about what you said. It was a totally new ballgame for me and it's still an issue in St. Anthony. Confidentiality among families wasn't something I had come across in the Britain. There, nobody knew anybody, so confidentiality wasn't an issue. In Forteau they were very inquisitive about me. I craved anonymity and still do sometimes. I missed it!

"Adapting to the long, bitter winter was another adjustment but my first winter was exciting. For three or four years winter was exciting, but then I reached a point when I hoped for good weather so I could travel back and forth to work. We moved to the community my husband was from, about nine miles outside Forteau. It was a 10 or 15 minute drive in summer, but it was a totally different ballgame in winter! When the weather was really bad we went by Ski-Doo, but many times I had to stay in Forteau overnight and couldn't get home to my two young children. That was another reason we moved to St. Anthony. We said we wanted a place on the doorstep of the hospital so weather wouldn't be an issue. Now I can see the hospital from my living room window.

"One of the nurses in Forteau had been there since the mid '50s, and when she came it was quite primitive, with dog teams, and had very little electricity. I read about Labrador before I came, but the material was obviously out of date because I was amazed at how advanced it was. The roads were gravel but people had deep freezers, dishwashers, and their houses were absolutely beautiful. Also the standard of living was much higher than where I had lived in the east end of London. It was an area with a lot of poverty and a lot of immigrants. Also poverty in a city is quite different from poverty in a rural area. Forteau was not affluent but had more amenities than I expected and was more comfortable. People had gardens but I missed fresh milk. A few people had cows but I didn't like the milk because I was used to pasteurized milk, so we used canned milk.

"There was a nurse in Forteau nearing retirement who had an incredible bank of knowledge and another nurse from England. They were really my mentors for the first year. The nursing station was a big house. In the basement was a little pharmacy with a little wicket door, a waiting room and two clinic rooms. Upstairs was a kitchen, dining room, and two rooms for overnight patients who couldn't get out to St. Anthony hospital. A doctor came from Flower's Cove for three or four days every four to six weeks. But doctors in St. Anthony were only a phone call away. Also the two experienced outpost nurses were as good as any doctor and always knew which patients to send out and which ones to hang on to.

"Forteau had a radio system with a call signal. Every morning we radioed the patients' status into the head nurse in St. Anthony. They told us who was coming home and asked if we could send in patients who needed surgery. We phoned around to see who could find a babysitter so they could go for their surgery. That only happened for a year.

"We lived and worked in the nursing station so it was 24/7! We even worked on your so-called day off if it got busy. We were never away from work! On your days off you'd hear the telephone ringing because the sound-proofing was very poor. And you could hear patients talking to each other in the waiting room.

"We had a patient with MS who lived in the nursing station, and we'd get up to help turn this lady whether we were working or not. When the clinic opened this lady was re-located to a long-term care facility in Blanc Sablon in Quebec. She wasn't French but it was a special arrangement so she was within travelling distance for her family to visit. That was so sad! We were close to the Quebec border. If the weather was down and we couldn't send a patient to St. Anthony we often sent them to the hospital in Blanc Sablon.

"They were laying the foundation for the new Health Centre when I arrived in Forteau. It was obvious things were going to change, and they did big time! When we moved into the clinic we had to find our own accommodations, but after a year of living and working in the same building I was ready to get out of there because you never escaped work.

"We went from three to five nurses and had a full-time family doctor in the community which made a big difference. In some ways we were less reliant on St. Anthony, but with the doctor came more referrals to St. Anthony. Also there were more diagnostic procedures being done and technologies like scanners and ultrasound were coming on line. We had holding beds in the clinic but weren't allowed to admit patients any longer than a night or two. They were very strict about that because we didn't live in the clinic. If we had inpatients and the nurse got called out at night we had to call in another nurse. That was a very expensive way of caring for them.

"I travelled by plane in winter and by road in summer. We went to Red Bay once a week for clinic and that took about an hour and a half on a very poor dirt road. We saw between 30 and 35 patients and whoever was really sick came back to Forteau in a four-wheel drive. Shortly after the new clinic opened, they paved the road. Those weekly clinics stopped and patients from Red Bay came to Forteau. That was one of many politically unpopular decisions that were made.

"I worked as a community midwife and outpost nurse in Forteau. We booked everyone for delivery because then, the women went to St. Anthony for delivery and we didn't do home deliveries. We delivered undiagnosed twins in the nursing station at 34 weeks. It was quite exciting, but I'll never forget it! We sent them to St. Anthony and they did well. Also there were women who engineered it so they didn't go out. We had one or two who dug in their heels and wouldn't go until they had pain, and by then it was too late to send them out.

"I spent six years in Labrador and during that time I met my husband and got married. Once our children came along, there were certain things about living and working in the same community. The pressure was not always a good thing and it was difficult to get away from work. At home the phone was always ringing, even on my day off. People would ask, 'Do you think I should go to clinic?' and in order to answer you had to hear the whole spiel. Also, I wanted my kids to grow up in a bigger centre and I missed working in a hospital. I didn't want to work in the clinic for the rest of my life. My husband was happy to move to St. Anthony. We knew the town and he had family there. I worked as a midwife at the hospital for three or four years then went into the operating room because it was a Monday to Friday job. I thought I'd give it a try and I loved it and have been there ever since. That was a big switch!

"People said I was adaptable, but I didn't think of myself that way. I relished change and every two or three years I needed something different to do. I did that until I was almost 40, then decided I didn't like change quite as much. Going to the OR was a good thing because it came at a time when I wanted a challenge and it was very positive and stimulating for me.

"My children are grown, but I find it hard to accept that both have gone to the mainland like a lot of Newfoundland children. Mine went there after high school for their education. They liked it there and stayed. Also their partners are there, so it is unlikely they will come back.

"I've kept in touch with my relatives in Britain, and over the years all of my family have been here. Now we meet in Canada as much as we do in Britain. They love where we are. For them this is a real holiday and break from Britain where it is very crowded. I always say the difference between Newfoundland and Britain is the number of people. Imagine Newfoundland with 59 million people on the island; that's what England is like. I never felt I wanted to go back. I enjoyed my holidays in England, but I've always enjoyed living here. As time moves on I'm glad this is where I settled."

❧

Margaret (Maggie) (Arkell) Linstead was born in Hitchin, England. She graduated from St. Bartholomew's Hospital in London as a SRN in 1979. She completed midwifery and graduated as a Registered Midwife from Norwich Hospital in Norwich, Norfolk, in 1981. That same year she came to work at the Forteau nursing station.

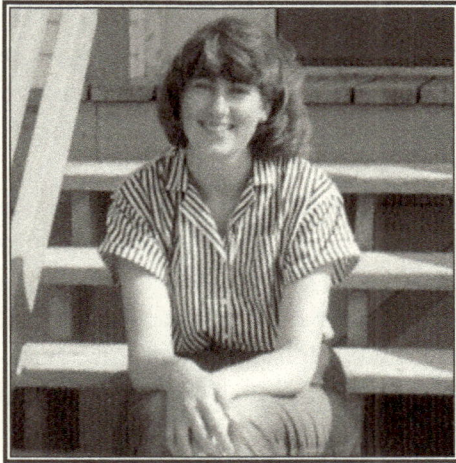

KAREN (FLINT) DYKE

❀

1988

"Two weeks after I arrived I was asked to go to Cartwright temporarily because there was no nurse there. I had no idea what I was getting into! But after I settled, I decided I'd stay."

"I always liked travelling so after I did midwifery I thought I'd go someplace like Africa, but you had to sign a two-year contract, which I didn't want to do. Grenfell was recruiting at the time so I came to Labrador. They had an ad in a nursing magazine and set up videos and displays in a London hotel. They showed pictures of Nain, which they described as a cottage hospital with six nurses and a doctor. Everything looked lovely! I decided that's what I'd do.

"There was a lot of paperwork to immigrate. I applied to the Canadian High Commission in London for a work permit and had to renew my passport. Grenfell advised me how to speed things up, but they were limited because I just had to go through the process. The paperwork was in place in November so I thought, 'That's it, just go on!' I came on a temporary licence and wrote the Canadian RN exam in January after I started working in Cartwright. Grenfell flew me to St. John's to sit the exam.

"The pay was better here than in London then. Even now Canadian nurses are paid better than English nurses. I came on a one-year contract and wasn't planning to be here for 17 years! Grenfell paid my way here and would pay my way back when I fulfilled the year.

"I flew to St. John's and Grenfell had told me to phone when I arrived. The hospital plane wasn't in so they said to go to the Airport Inn. I paid for that and Grenfell looked after me. They arranged a commercial flight to St. Anthony for six o'clock the next morning. It was a bit nerve-wracking to see this little 10-seat plane. St. Anthony seemed like a nice small town. There was only a small hall and a cinema, but people were very nice. One of the nurses was very good to me and made sure I had the proper winter clothing. Grenfell didn't tell you about clothes before you came. The recruiter in London suggested I get clothing here and not buy something in London that wasn't suitable for here because winters here are totally different from England!

"I stayed in St. Anthony in a Grenfell apartment for a week or two for orientation. It was a general orientation to the hospital and I met the doctors, so I'd be familiar with the kind of patients to expect. It was mostly meeting the people I'd be talking to about patients. It's hard to talk to someone over the phone but it helps if you've met them. Two weeks after I arrived I was asked to go to Cartwright temporarily because there was no nurse there. I had no idea what I was getting into! But after I settled, I decided to stay.

"I flew on a little plane from St. Anthony and stopped in all the communities from there to Goose Bay, which was six or seven stops. Cartwright was the last but one. That was nerve-wracking because I didn't know where I was. Black Tickle is just before Cartwright and there the plane backs around so all you see is rock and ground. Then, being November, the further north we went the more snow and ice there was. I'm wondering, 'What am I doing here?'

"After nursing school I worked in the x-ray department doing mostly radiology. I worked on a medical floor only a few months before I did midwifery. Then I worked a year in midwifery so my acute care experience was limited. But I thought people in England and Canada have the same complaints: colds, flu and that kind of stuff. Also I always thought nursing is 50 percent common sense, and if you have that things will be okay. Seventeen years later I think, 'Oh my gosh! What did I do that for?'

"There were two nurses in Cartwright from Flower's Cove. They stayed the weekend to give me an overview and left on Monday. A supervisor flew from St. Anthony that evening and stayed a week. Cartwright was supposed to have two nurses but they had a recruitment problem so initially I was there alone.

"The people of Cartwright were very excited about my arrival and very pleased to meet me. It was funny! They made appointments to come in with their complaints so then they could say they'd met the new nurse. Cartwright is in a small bay and the Grenfell clinic was on one side and the town on the other. We were apart from the main town but joined in activities. We were probably under the spotlight more than we realized.

"The clinic got a lot of phone calls, but I couldn't answer the phone because I couldn't understand what people were saying, so I'd pass it to the nursing aides. In England there are different dialects, but in Newfoundland there are a lot of differences. It was terribly difficult for me at first. I didn't find it too bad face-to-face, but sometimes people spoke faster than I was used to. But usually the nursing aide was around and she was really good. She knew everybody, which was half of it. A woman brought in her son and said he had a problem with his bird. I had no idea what that meant. She pulled up his shirt, so I thought she meant the belly button, but then she started to pull down his pants and I figured out what the problem was!

"I didn't have difficulty adapting to the names of the medications. If there was something on a medication I didn't recognize, I looked it up. I was in-charge in Cartwright and was responsible for ordering pharmacy supplies, so I got to know the names of things. I found differences between Canadian and English nursing. The hospitals here are set up differently with single or four-bed rooms, whereas the hospitals in London where I trained had open wards. The nursing hierarchy here is better; it's more open. As a student in England you had Sister who was in-charge and staff nurses, and they weren't always approachable. The charge nurses I've worked with here have been very friendly and open and encourage questions. There is more equality among staff here. I've always found people here very friendly and they go out of their way to help.

"Cartwright had a big clinic. It had been a hospital but was renovated. People were upset about losing their hospital. The nursing staff lived upstairs. On the middle floor was the clinic, a large nurses' room with an examination room off that, a little pharmacy, and the doctors' room. There were two rooms, one with a bed and a cot and the other had two beds. Downstairs was the dental area, the public health nurse's office, a small waiting room along with the laundry room and maintenance room. We had a maintenance man on staff who did call, and two nursing aides—one worked during the day and the other came in the evening and when clinic was busy. There were another three or four nursing aides who I could call if needed. An Irish nurse came in January or February and the public health nurse started when I did. She was based in Cartwright and travelled to Goose Bay, Black Tickle, and Mary's Harbour.

"The doctor came from St. Anthony or Goose Bay. Our doctor was a native Labradorian, based in Goose Bay, so she knew everybody. The dentist flew in but didn't come very often. We lost the dentist the summer after I came, so we had to send people out. Others, like the ophthalmologist and physio, travelled through periodically. That was different because I worked in a big London hospital and had the support of colleagues, senior staff, and doctors. Also equipment and everything was at hand. In a nursing station you're alone and have to deal with things as they happen. I could call the doctor if I had any questions, but occasionally I had to arrange for patients to go out.

I was called to an accident one night. Two people, who were drunk on a Ski-Doo, hit a rock and went flying. They came to the clinic. One had a head injury. I called the doctor and arranged a flight out for the morning, so I stayed with them all night. The phone kept ringing, so I called in a nursing aide because you can only do so much yourself. I only kept people overnight if I had to. There weren't many night calls, which was good, because I don't do well with sleep deprivation. The people appreciated my time and didn't get me up if they didn't have to. If I was called at night the maintenance man came with me because I didn't know where anybody lived. He had a big GM truck and we'd load a stretcher in the back. There was a hook in the ceiling for an IV bag. Usually we brought the person back to the clinic.

"Restructuring of health care happened just after I left. Although while I was there, one of the administrators from St. Anthony brought two people from the mainland into all the communities to have meetings about what people wanted. Bringing in outsiders was a waste of time! I was there less than a year and could have told them what the issues were. Anybody in the community could have told them! But there wasn't a lot of community consultation, which was disappointing. One issue for Cartwright was the name of their clinic. They wanted to call it after a nurse who had been in the community when the hospital was there, but St. Anthony wanted to call it something else. There was a bit of wrangling over that! There was a committee with myself and people of the community which reported to St. Anthony, and the clinic's name was always on the agenda! I thought they should be able to call the clinic what they wanted because it was their community and they had lost their hospital.

"You made your own fun. We joined in community activities like broomball games. We also had volleyball, bingo, and the usual activities at Christmas. We were always invited to these things.

"I left Cartwright because I had enough of the isolation and really didn't get on with my supervisor. I went home that Easter to my friend's wedding and met my husband in Cartwright when I came back, so I had to decide what to do next. I had a job in a nursing station in Ontario but didn't take it. I worked in Goose Bay in the midwifery unit for two months but that wasn't a permanent move. Meeting my husband influenced my decision to go there because I wanted to work in the province. Otherwise, I was moving on. It's just the way things seemed to fall!

"We planned to get married, but my work permit expired and I wasn't able to renew it so I couldn't work. We bought a house together and I was able to go back to work after I got married. It wasn't a difficult decision to stay. It was probably more difficult for my parents. They didn't say anything and certainly wouldn't discourage me. They were happy because I was happy. I go home every couple of years and they come over. It helps being able to get back and forth.

"I wouldn't go back to England to live. My son is 12 and wouldn't live anywhere else. My husband is a true Newfoundlander and wouldn't even consider living on the mainland. Apart from my family, there isn't much for me in England now. The health system has changed so much, and I wouldn't get a position at the pay scale I would want, even with my experience. Also to buy property there is horrendous, and to some extent the cost of living and the lifestyle. Here we have a good-sized home on a good lot and we're settled. St. John's has plenty of cultural and other activities if you want and traffic isn't bad. My career here has been interesting and varied. I've never gotten a negative response from the nurses I've worked with. They're always fascinated with my accent and accept me as a colleague."

❋

Karen (nee Flint) Dyke was born in London, England. She graduated in 1984 as a RGN in general nursing from Whittington Hospital, Highgate, London. She completed an 18-month midwifery program as a SCM at Northwich Park, Harrow, England, in 1986. She immigrated to work at the nursing station in Cartwright in 1988.

Chapter Five

ST. ANTHONY

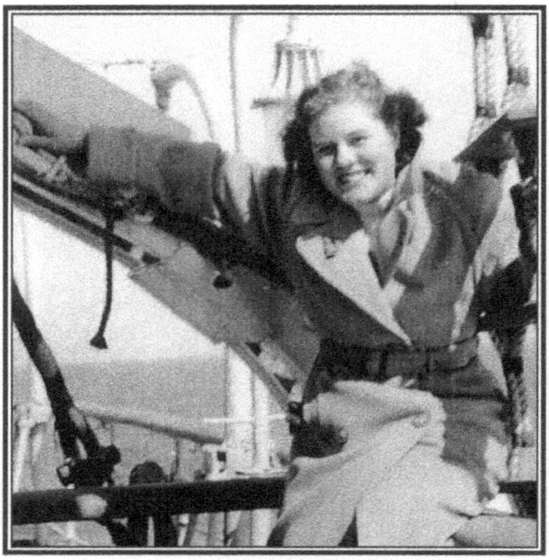

SHEILA (FORTESCUE) PADDON

1949

"It's hard to describe what it was like in present-day terms because it was a different world ... We looked after people and that was our life."

"Nurses couldn't leave England for a year after the war, which was part of government's plan because Britain needed nurses. I worked in London briefly as a midwife before I decided to come work in Labrador with the Grenfell mission. I knew about it because as children we put pennies in missionary boxes for Dr. Grenfell. Also I knew people who worked in Labrador and enjoyed it. Grenfell had two contracts: one for volunteers who worked six months with no pay and paid their own passage over, and another for four years where you got paid. I came in 1949 as a volunteer because I wasn't sure I'd be suitable.

"I came to St. John's by boat and was met by the secretary of the Grenfell missions. I was going to St. Anthony by boat but the *Kyle* was ice-bound. I stayed at the old Newfoundland Hotel and heard a plane was flying to St. Anthony with a part for the fish plant. It was a float plane and somebody said maybe I could fly up and I did. We stopped overnight in Roddickton and I stayed with a family because the nursing station was full. We went to St. Anthony the next day, but it was ice-bound so the pilot landed in St. Anthony Byte.

"I lived in the hospital which had the nurses' bedrooms and bathrooms on one side. On the other was a ward, the OR, a sterilizing room, x-ray, and offices were in the centre. There was a dining room where everybody ate and a sitting room for the nurses.

"I worked in St. Anthony six months and loved every moment. It was demanding and busy with only four nurses, but I thought it was a great life. The hospital had 80 beds and two doctors. The nurses did general nursing and deliveries but they had midwifery training. Grenfell had a barn with cows and sometimes I did the milking because I had done dairy farming before I went into nursing. The *Kyle* brought patients from the coast and TB patients who were sick. There was a lot of TB. There were nursing stations in Cartwright, Mary's River, Mary's Harbour, Forteau, and Flower's Cove, and the nurses there were on their own. Occasionally they saw a doctor to discuss patients' problems, and that summer a doctor set up a RT so the nurses could call in and we could call out.

"It's hard to describe what it was like in present-day terms because it was a different world. We were there as nurses and we nursed. We looked after people and that was our life. We did whatever came to hand. We didn't have a social life; you never thought of it and we didn't go there for that. There was no such thing as time off, but if we weren't busy some went off for a bit. I went for walks in my free time. Occasionally, when we weren't busy, whoever could be spared went on the mission motorboat for an hour or two.

Come from Away

NURSES WHO IMMIGRATED TO NEWFOUNDLAND AND LABRADOR

"At the end of my six months they asked me to stay and open Spotted Island, which was closed during the war, but I had to go home. The mission staff travelled on the SS *Newfoundland* and SS *Nova Scotia*, two ships that went back and forth to Liverpool. I told my family I enjoyed my stay and was going back. They wanted to know where I was going and I said, 'It's in Labrador. It's a great life and suits me very well.' I had done midwifery part one and thought I'd finish part two before I returned, because that was the practical where you got experience doing deliveries alone. When I finished I took a few months to do deliveries until I knew enough to go to a nursing station alone.

"When I returned I wasn't prepared to sign on for four years, so I agreed to come for one and decide later. Grenfell only agreed because they needed nurses. North West River needed a nurse because the nurse had been there for six years with few breaks and hadn't been home to England in that time. I flew back because there was a flight from London to Goose Bay then. Nobody gave you directions, but it was post-war and everything was disorganized. I was just told to come to Goose Bay. We landed in the middle of the night. I wandered outside and into a cemetery but eventually came back to a big building and found a bed. It was a barracks because there was a large air force complement in Goose Bay then. Eventually they woke me and took me to Happy Valley in a truck.

"Happy Valley was a tiny nursing station with one nurse and two beds. It was an old building given to the Grenfell mission by the air force. The nurse said the boat would come from North West River for me but she didn't know when. It seems strange now, but that's how it was then and that was the charm of it. Anyway, I got to North West River and the nurse was anxious to leave. She told me about the patients, their diagnoses, and treatments and that Dr. Paddon was there but leaving the next day. She showed me the RT and other things then said, 'I have to go to get the plane,' and left!

"I was alone in North West River and thought it was wonderful because I had my own hospital. It was supposed to have eight or 10 beds, but beds were everywhere, along with children's cots. There was a dispensary and a Benfell chair in a corner, which was the dentist office. There was a table with test tubes and a few bobbits and an x-ray machine. Dr. Paddon's father had worked with Dr. Grenfell and built the first hospital in North West River but died suddenly in '39. His wife ran the hospital during the war and his son returned there after serving in the war. I fit in very well. I was busy but didn't have time to think about it. North West River was different from St. Anthony because the doctor travelled a lot and I had all the responsibility. Grenfell had a hospital ship called the *Maraval* with an x-ray on board. Every summer she went to White Bay and around the northern Newfoundland coast to St. Anthony, then she crossed the straits to North West River and up to Hebron looking for TB and things. The doctor went on the *Maraval* for several weeks, so people on the coast saw the doctor once each summer and once each winter when he went by dog team. Otherwise there were only the nurses in Hopedale and Makkovik.

"I had two aides from North West River who were very good. One could tell spot on if it was time to deliver a patient. She'd send a boy with a note, because there were no telephones, asking, 'Could I come please?' The other nurse trained them. They spoke a little Inuktitut, but there weren't as many northern people living here then. They only came down the coast if they were sick. We had Inuit people across the river who came every spring, put up tents, and stayed for the summer. Then suddenly one day in the fall, they'd be gone to live in-country all winter. We were busy when they came because many got injured during the winter, but they looked after themselves very well, far better than we did sometimes. We had a boy with a severe dog bite on his leg. We did a skin graft, which was doing well, but the time came for his people to move back to the country. His father walked into the hospital, put the boy over his shoulder and walked out. I worried the leg wouldn't set and the skin grafts would be for nothing, but when they came back the following spring it was healed perfectly, better than we could have done. That kind of thing made it interesting. You pulled on all your resources, which was good because that's how it was.

"After four months leave, the nurse returned to North West River and I went to Harrington Harbour for the winter. It was in Quebec but had a Grenfell hospital. Getting there was a problem because you weren't given instructions, just told, 'Go to so-and-so.' If you didn't mind that sort of thing, it was a great life. Somebody flew me to Seven Islands on the Quebec shore then said, 'This is as far as we take you, but there is a boat,' which was the last one for the season! There was nobody else on the boat except the bishop of Quebec, who was a dear. He was visiting convents along the coast, and each time he visited the nuns I went with him to get supplies, a meal and a bath. They were wonderful! It was several days before we arrived at Harrington Harbour, which had a fairly new hospital but was a bleak and rocky place with no trees.

"The doctor there was Canadian. The two nurses left on the previous boat so there were no nurses in the hospital and they hadn't left things in a good state. The hospital was full and busy and the aides were caring for the patients. Many patients spoke French but also a little English. There was a lot of TB. The dentist had also gone but blessed us with a dental office. The doctor was so thankful I got there because he was going by dog team to visit communities down the north shore. I stayed the winter and it was a great experience!

"The Grenfell mission had industrial workers who did handicrafts like hooked rugs, and there was one worker from St. Anthony at the hospital. The housekeeper had left too, so the worker and I did house-keeping and nursing. Occasionally, I went by dog team to visit patients who were a distance away and had to decide whether they should come to hospital or not. There was supposed to be two nurses on staff but I never got a second one. The doctor in St. Anthony would say on the RT,

'Keep going, I'll find a nurse, don't worry!' I kept going but another nurse never materialized.

"Two nurses came to Harrington Harbour that spring and I went back to North West River because most of my things were there. Then Dr. Paddon and I got engaged so I went home to tell my family. My sister thought it strange and wanted to know who this man was. But my father said, 'You know what you're doing.' Everybody was very cheerful about it. I returned to get married in June, but the nurse in North West River left and I had to work. We still weren't married in September so we decided to get married one Saturday. Everybody in the community came and they gave us a wonderful party. But that night we were busy with a patient so we didn't get settled for a while. Finally a nurse came and I handed the hospital over to her and that was that!

"I didn't nurse or do midwifery after I married but they would call me if they needed assistance. Also, there were times when there was no nurse and I filled in. It was a great life because you were left alone. There weren't the tiresome regulations there are now. You used your common sense and good training and that's what it was about. When we built the new hospital in North West River, the Department of Health was involved and things changed. There were two nurses then and I only got called if they needed another pair of hands.

"Every four years IGA doctors got a sabbatical where they went out for six months in the winter. They went on the last boat of the year and returned on the first boat in the spring. It was a chance to catch up on medicine. My husband did surgery and dentistry at the hospital. He did a lot of TB chest and pulmonary drainage work so he did several months of surgery at the Mary Hitchcock Hospital in New England. Four years later he went to Miller Fields in London and did eyes. He also went to the Bond, a chest hospital in London to catch up on TB, although we had streptomycin by then. Before that TB was hopeless. The family went also and we rented a house. We had four children and I had to find schools for two of them. As soon as the ice went, usually in June, we had to return to North West River, but English schools didn't break up until August. We had to take the children out because they were little and we couldn't leave them. At one point we had four going to different boarding schools which took planning because some were in England and some in Canada, but the children took it in their stride.

"Grenfell ran dormitories so children from the coast could go to school. They had to come to North West River but only if the parents requested it. About 70 children came when school started in the fall and stayed until the spring. They were all ages and a mixture of all cultures, but mostly, they were children of white settlers on the coast. The Inuit and Indian children didn't come because they were in-country with their people. Some came from very isolated places and missed their families but after the first few days they had a great time because children love to be with other children. They were well cared for, had good food and surroundings and all sorts of entertainment. We had movies, and the men on the air force base had wonderful parties and games for them. I don't think it was much of a hardship for the children. We seldom had a child who was utterly miserable and wanting to go home. Some stayed from the time they started school until grade 11.

"The staff in the dormitories was House Mothers, most of whom came from England for two or three years but some stayed for years. They were wonderful women and great fun. The dormitories are closed now, but children who stayed there greet me on the road and say, 'Do you remember me? I was in the dorm!' Quite a few of the nurses who worked in North West River came from England. Most went home although some are still here. We had very few Newfoundland nurses because they didn't come here in those days and they didn't have the midwifery training, which was important.

"Grenfell used to be known as a mission but it isn't a mission anymore. Only the old ones like me remember that. In the early days, young people came to the mission every summer from the States to work as volunteers. They were called WOPs, which meant 'without pay.' For young people who wanted to go somewhere and do something interesting, working in Labrador was a good thing. Some summers we'd have 15 to 20 girls and boys, and this was a problem because they lived all over the place.

"I can't remember that I had a problem with the accent but it's been so long. The people here were great and so kind and good to the nurses. I'm happy I came to Newfoundland and happy I was a nurse. I'm glad I learned about Dr. Grenfell and the Grenfell Mission and that I met my husband here. I had a wonderful nursing experience here, which might not appeal to everyone, but having sole responsibility of a small hospital was for me a great undertaking. But I was well-trained, having nursed through the war, the bombing, and the blitz, and I knew midwifery. The people were so good and still are; they accepted me. I've lived in North West River since 1951 and our children came and went. My brother and his wife and my sister also visited. I'm still here and I'm home. I wouldn't live anywhere else."

※

Sheila (nee Fortescue) Paddon was born in Essex, England, and graduated as a SRN in 1944 from The Prince of Wales General Hospital in London. She completed midwifery Part 1 at Bearsted Hospital, London, before coming to St. Anthony as a volunteer nurse for six months in 1949. She returned to England to complete midwifery, Part 2 as a SCM, before returning in 1951 to work in North West River. She married Dr. Anthony Paddon, who was Lieutenant Governor of Newfoundland and Labrador from 1981 to 1986.

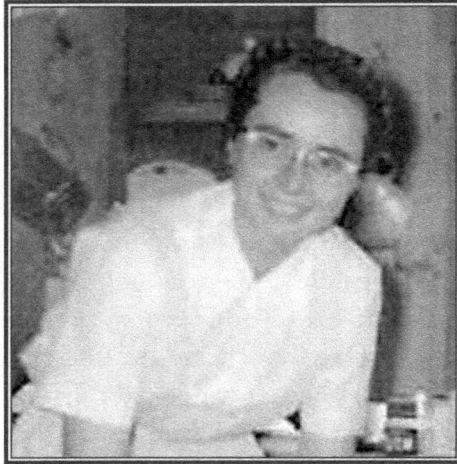

JEANETTE HOSTETER

✳

1957

*"I like it here. It's nice and peaceful and you can go out
in nature for walks and it's relatively safe. You can walk around
outside and not be afraid of being mugged."*

"I came to Newfoundland and Labrador through the Mennonite Central Committee, which is a church organization. They sent nurses, teachers, and doctors to areas where there was a need. I went to Twillingate for six weeks to do summer relief, then I came to St. Anthony.

"I flew into Gander in the middle of the night and went to Twillingate by way of Lewisporte. A lady and her children were also going there, so we shared a taxi. When we got to Lewisporte, the hotel had a room for the woman and her children. I had forgotten the name of my hotel so they put me in a room with somebody I didn't know, which was how they did it then. This other person was asleep so I crawled into the empty bed. Whoever it was was gone when I got up, so I never knew who I spent my first night with in Newfoundland! The next morning we took the boat to Twillingate because the road or causeway wasn't there then. It was a beautiful day when I arrived. I remember the lilacs were blooming because that was July and lilacs were over in Pennsylvania. The old hospital was on an unpaved road and everything was very dusty. That was my first impression! Twillingate was different, but I'm a country girl so I didn't find the smallness of the community strange.

"People showed me around the hospital and I went to work right away but I worked with somebody. The nurses here did more in the hospital like they were expected to deliver a baby. I only observed deliveries in nursing school so I didn't get involved in them at first, although I did deliveries when I got to St. Anthony. Some nurses in Twillingate trained at my school so I knew them, which helped. Also a couple in the community was like a mother and father to us so we spent a lot of time with them.

"When I was little I heard stories about missionaries who went places and thought I'd do that when I got older. I read about Grenfell in high school and thought Labrador would be good because usually they sent people to hot countries and I can't stand the heat. I had friends who worked in Newfoundland with the Mennonite Central Committee and thought I'd apply because there was a real shortage of nurses here. When I applied, the Mennonites weren't sending people to St. Anthony but told me they would be, so I thought, 'I'll go to St. Anthony.' The hospital plane picked up a group in Gander then me in Twillingate. It was a float plane and there were three nurses, a teacher, and a doctor on the plane.

"The Mennonite Central Committee paid my way in and out. It was a volunteer program so I got room and board and spending money every month. We got $10,000 in the first year, $20,000 in the second year, and that money went to the Committee who sent it to support the

Albert Schweitzer Hospital in Haiti.

"The nurses shared a room in an area of the old hospital called the nurses' corridor, which was connected to the San. We had a sitting room downstairs where we gathered in the evenings for tea. We had a dining room, which was cafeteria style, but they had a buffet and we served our own meals. We had a coffee break each morning and tea each afternoon but only if you could run to the living room! Sometimes we had cookies and one cook occasionally made Baked Alaska, which was a special treat. He still lives here and when I see him I always ask if he remembers those beautiful Baked Alaskas and he does!

"When we arrived in St. Anthony, the nurses were so glad because they had help. The head nurse actually said, 'I'll be able to give the girls a day off now.' They needed somebody in the operating room (OR) and the other nurses wouldn't go so I said, 'I haven't done surgery since nursing school,' which had been five years, but they said, 'That's all right, you can learn,' so I went. The nurse there might have spent a day with me before she moved to the wards and I was left with two aides who were very good. I stayed there for two years.

"I didn't have difficulty with the language except when people added or subtracted the h's. Also they spoke very fast so I had to say, 'Speak a little slower!' At the hospital they used English terminology like theatre for operating room or trolley for stretcher. They'd say, 'Take the trolley to the theatre.' Eventually I began to think on the same wavelength. I was North American and most of the other nurses here were English.

"I was in the OR one stormy night when we got a message that a lady in Cook's Harbour was having a baby but having trouble. In those days there was no telephone, only the telegram. When we finished working, a couple of doctors decided to go there on the big snowmobile we had then, which had a red cross on it. Meanwhile, the people from Cook's Harbour decided to fly the lady in. One doctor and a nurse who did anesthetics had stayed at the hospital and decided to do a section. Another nurse and I were also there. It was a difficult case because the woman bled a lot. The others got back and scrubbed in and we got a live baby and mother. They did rounds the next morning and the woman was in bed eating grapes! I saw her years later and asked if she remembered that night and she said, 'Oh yes!'

"After that I worked on the wards. There was a unit, which was a TB San, and two general wards, with obstetrics included, called Gen 1 and Gen 2. There was one RN on evenings and nights, and they covered the whole hospital after 7:00 p.m. with aides on each floor. There were about 100 patients in the San who stayed a long time and about 50 patients on the other floors. I also worked with OBS. If we weren't busy in the OR, we covered labour and delivery.

"On the wards we got two half days off a week: Saturday afternoons and a half day on Sundays. Every six weeks or so we might get a day off if there was enough people. We walked a lot because there were great places to walk. There was no television so we created our own entertainment. A doctor who was a good singer came from England for one winter. We didn't have much time, but we managed to do a couple of shows for the community in the high school auditorium. We even took it to Flower's Cove—just put the piano in the back of the truck! There was a movie theatre in town and the hospital had entertainment. There was a US base when I came and people went to see movies there. Also, people sang in church choirs or were involved with the schools. Unfortunately I wasn't a singer. I'm Mennonite but I worshipped at the United Church and still go there.

"Grenfell's boat, the *Maravel*, visited the nursing stations because doctors didn't go there often. A doctor and the nurse from the nursing station went to communities in the area. I did the ophthalmology course, we did eye clinics on the boat, which wasn't very satisfactory because even anchored the boat rocked, and it was difficult to examine eyes. Eventually we did eye clinics in the school or nursing station. When we used the float plane to do eye clinics, we had to load equipment into a small boat to get it into the community. When we took patients on the

Maraval or the float plane they came out in small boats and if they were really sick they were on stretchers. It was hard getting them up the steps from the small boat. You had to be very agile!

"I've been in St. Anthony 50 years with a few breaks every now and again. I went to Boston to do an OBS course then to Baie Verte cottage hospital for about nine months. Then I went to Toronto for a practical experience in ophthalmology and did a working holiday in England for nine months.

"I have a sister-in-law and niece in North Carolina and a nephew in Pennsylvania, so one year I go to North Carolina and the next go to Pennsylvania. I went there every year when my parents were there but they didn't visit here. They weren't much for travelling, but when they were too old to travel, I think they wished they had come. When I told my mother I was going away, she said, 'I have a feeling you're going to stay because a lot of people who travel stay away.' I remember saying, 'I don't think so. I'll come back after a year. I'm not like those people!' But I don't think my parents were surprised when I came back here. We always kept in contact, but first when I came it was letters because there was no telephone.

"Initially I came to Newfoundland for a year and extended to three. I went home for six months and came back on staff at St. Anthony hospital. I like it here. It's nice and peaceful and you can go out in nature for walks and it's relatively safe. You can walk outside and not be afraid of being mugged."

❋

Jeanette Hosteter was born in Lancaster, Pennsylvania, and graduated in 1952 with an RN diploma from Lancaster General Hospital. In 1957 she came to Twillingate for six weeks as a volunteer with the Mennonite Central Committee. From there she went to St. Anthony.

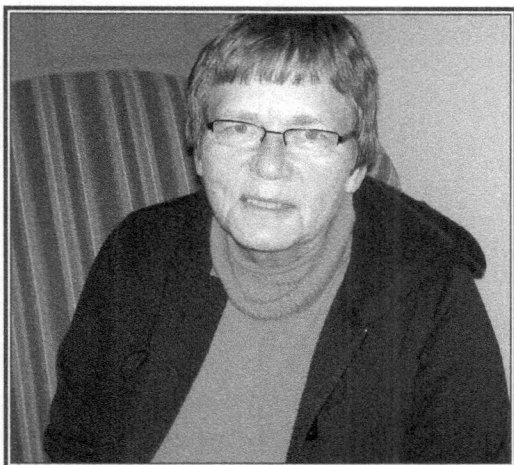

JANE JOHANNSEN

✿

1975

"In the beginning the people in the community put me up on a pedestal because I was a nurse. I think it was because we helped them when they had hardships so they knew they could trust us."

"I worked as a nursing assistant in the casualty department in a hospital in Stockholm but got tired of that and went to England to do my SRN and SCM. During the midwifery program I was in the library and found Grenfell's book. The story stayed with me as something I'd like to do. When I finished midwifery I decided to come. I didn't have a problem getting registered, although it took time to get everything in order, but the Grenfell people helped.

"I didn't know what to expect when I came, but I thought, 'It can't be too bad because other people have done it.' I landed in Gander and the hospital plane picked me up. When we landed in St. Anthony, a man came over and asked, 'Are you Jane?' The Grenfell bus drove me into town. Three or four nurses shared an apartment and the rent was subsidized. We each had a bedroom and you cooked for yourself. Everybody was very helpful and I thought, 'I owe these people a lot.' The salary wasn't much but I came for the adventure. I don't recall if they paid my way here but later when they were short of nurses they did offer incentives.

"I worked in pediatrics at St. Anthony hospital. I never worked on the coast although I did do medevacs. I arrived one day, went to work the next, got my patient assignment and that was it! The head nurse gave me a little orientation and that was about all there was. You weren't given time to adjust to the environment. Comparing nursing practice at Grenfell with my experience in London, I would say everybody here was very professional. That amazed me because I thought I was coming to the boonies and that things might be a little lax, but the nurses here were very professional. It took them a while to figure out I was an odd person, and we did have differences but nothing major. When I was a head nurse I thought things should be done my way because it was my responsibility, but not everybody agreed. I liked things my way and I think I did a good job.

"After four years on peds, I went head nurse in ICU for four or five years. That was very interesting! I did a medevac to Nain to pick up a lady who was in jail there. I think she had something cardiac. I went to the jail and the police were there. She needed an IV but fought at all turns, so we strapped her down. She had a few choice words for us! We flew her out and it was hard caring for a patient in an aircraft, especially one who didn't want to be there. My thinking on medevacs was that we should do what we could, then get the patient to the hospital. But others thought you should keep trying to stabilize rather than get the patient on the plane and out. The pilot did radio in to where we were going, but we didn't always have radio contact so you couldn't always tell them what you were doing for the patient. We also medevaced babies to the Janeway. We did medevacs alone, although if it was a baby we had two people, but not always two nurses.

"I had a patient from Goose Bay who had lung problems and very poor breathing, but he wouldn't stop smoking. We battled daily to see who would win about his smoking because he had a mind of his own. He didn't speak English so we also had a problem understanding each other. He'd have a slew of visitors every day, and I'd hear them talking and see them pointing at me. But after a while we began to understand each other and things got better.

"We had a lot of babies, but I liked looking after them. It was a good challenge until you lost one and you'd always think, 'What did I do wrong?' Also, you'd think about their family. We had three sisters as patients; the oldest was 16 and they died one after the other from a breathing problem. That was so hard. Most patients came from St. Anthony, but a lot came from the coast which was sad because their family couldn't visit. The families there were very close-knit and the patients needed them.

"After ICU, I was Director of Allied Health responsible for the professionals in physio, social work, and pharmacy. That was a challenge from the beginning because being supervised by a nurse was a sore issue. I gave them freedom to do things, as long as they could justify what they had done, and told them I'd only make changes if they were necessary. I thought I was fair but other people thought I was autocratic. I did that until I retired four years ago.

"I didn't have trouble adapting to the culture. I thrive on stuff like that. I preferred the people from the coast with problems like low income because I saw it as a challenge. I didn't have trouble with the local dialect but people had problems with my language. In the beginning people in the community put me on a pedestal because I was a nurse. I think it was because we helped them when they had hardships so they knew they could trust us. People were very friendly and invited us over or brought us a loaf of bread.

"I like nature and it's fantastic here because you can go into the outdoors. I liked the freedom of going into the hills and I liked skiing. Other than that, there wasn't a lot to do. The nurses gelled together and made our own entertainment. It was like a family. I stayed here because I liked the people I worked with and those I knew in town. I'm still in contact with friends in St. Anthony. At work I liked being part of a team and seeing things happening—although when we did restructuring in later years, it wasn't an easy time.

"My sister and her family are in Sweden, but she never came here. I visited in the beginning until my parents died. I retired here after 35 years' service, so what I call family is here. I wondered about going back to Denmark or Sweden but thought, 'I've more friends here than if I went home.' I went to Denmark last year to visit my aunt, thinking I might stay, but she died. Also there were so many changes. You expect things to be the same as when you left, and I went around trying to find places I remembered. I found my old school but it wasn't as I remembered it. I felt comfortable coming back here. Also I had no benefits in Sweden, so it was economically better for me to live here. My friends here were the biggest reason for coming back. My best memories of living in St. Anthony are feeling at peace and very much at home. I always felt looked after and safe in the community. I felt comfortable coming back."

❋

Jane Johannsen was born in Hastskovagen, Tyresol, Sweden. She graduated as a SRN from St. Olaves Hospital, London, England, in 1970. She completed a SCM from St. Helier Hospital in Carshalton, Surrey, England, and came to St. Anthony's hospital in 1975.

ARUNA THAMPY

✻

1975

*"I had no work expectations when I went to
the coast. I was told to work and I did. We worked
24 hours, six or six and half days a week,
and rarely got a day off."*

"I was working in England and a colleague showed me two advertisements in a midwifery journal: one for Singapore and one for IGA
looking for people to work with aboriginal people in northern Labrador.
I wrote to both and decided I'd go with whoever answered first. I heard
from IGA in London immediately and went for an interview. The office
had pictures of dog teams and I asked if they still had them and she said
yes. IGA got my ticket, visa, and everything done very quickly. I arrived
in Gander and called the RT office to find out when the IGA plane
would pick me up. They said, 'Find a hotel because the plane isn't
coming today. And keep in touch.' There were no hotel rooms because
there was a conference in town. I told the airport security guard because
I didn't know what to do. He put me in an airport room for maternity
mothers. The plane picked me up the next day. Dr. Thomas, his wife,
and mother were aboard and we went to St. John's. We arrived 10:00
a.m. Dr. Thomas told me not to leave the airport and be ready to leave

at 9:00 p.m. I stayed there for a bit then took a taxi tour of St. John's. The taxi driver said, 'I'll show you everything for $20.00,' and he did.

"When we got to St. Anthony airport, I was so excited because we drove in on a dirt road and I thought I was a pioneer! I understood I was coming to an outpost to work with the Inuit who lived in igloos. Driving from the airport they told me there were no dog teams. When we entered St. Anthony I was shocked to see a beautiful modern hospital in the middle of nowhere. It looked better than the hospital I trained in! The orientation nurse met me. When I asked where the Indians were, she thought it was funny and said they didn't have Indians anymore. I was extremely disappointed and didn't want to stay because I had come to nurse aboriginal people. But I thought 'I can't go home, so grin and bear it.'

"The Grenfell people in England asked me where I wanted to work and I said not geriatrics or pediatrics. When I arrived I was working on peds at the St. Anthony hospital. I was devastated! There were two pediatric units: neonatal to toddler, where I worked, and toddler upwards. The children came from the Labrador coast and the north shore of Quebec. The wards were always full. The children had sicknesses I'd never seen, like tetanus and kwashiorkor disease, which is a protein deficiency. I was amazed because I thought Canada was medically rich.

"After three weeks the head nurse put me on nights, but I didn't mind because the children slept and it wasn't as chaotic as days. I requested a transfer to outpatients but was denied. Kids came to hospital by plane with plasters attached to their clothes with their names on them. I asked where they came from and who put the tape on. The head nurse said, 'The outpost nurses.' I asked how to become one and she said, 'I don't think the Director of Nursing will let you go.'

"I came in June, and by July I was either going back to Kenya or to where these children came from.' So I said, 'Then I'll go home. Would you rather I stayed or leave?'

"I quickly realized the Grenfell people mixed and partied with their own. But I came for adventure and not to end up in little Britain. An Irish nurse and I partied with the local people; we ate nicer food and the people took us Ski-Dooing. It was fantastic. I had a wonderful time!

"I asked to be housed with a Canadian nurse. There were two Newfoundland nurses who wanted to show us how to make jam. They sent us to pick red berries and said how hard it was bending to pick them. We had a grand time and picking them had been easy. We picked tons and I called her at work to ask what to do and she said, 'Boil them.' We boiled and boiled and boiled! When she came home she died laughing because we picked dogberries not partridgeberries!

"Two colleagues applied for a position for me in Forteau but didn't tell me. The nursing director at the hospital who was filling in for the nursing director of nursing stations called me and said I wasn't suitable. I asked why and she said, 'It's a different culture. It's best to work here for six months. We gave you your visa to come and we can take it away.' I think IGA's recruitment strategy was to say you'd get the unit of your choice and then send you where the need was when you arrived. They paid my passage, so I was willing to stay a year if I went to an outpost. Otherwise I'd pay them back and go home. Somebody saw in my application that I was a midwife and Catholic, and decided to send me to Forteau. I had no idea religion meant so much in those days. The director at Curtis was not happy because she was losing a nurse from pediatrics. The following week I was asked to go to Forteau because they wanted to see if I would like it. I sat in the front of the aircraft and the pilot would descend to show me the whales and icebergs. What he didn't realize was that I was getting greener by the minute! The maintenance man took me to the station, but the nurse was busy in the orthopedic clinic and didn't know I was coming. She came up and said, 'Find a place to sit. Lunch is at 12:30. Don't be late!' I went to the kitchen to introduce myself and the cook said, 'We're not allowed to speak to the nurses.' I asked why and she said, 'That's the rule here.' It was a beautiful day so I took a blanket and went outside. I fell asleep on the hill and was late for lunch! The cook had put it aside but the nurse was not amused.

"This nurse had been there almost 28 years. After dinner she met with me and was very nice, but you could tell she didn't have any time for me. She'd had another nurse for 13 years, but she was sent to Flower's Cove although she didn't want to go. But in those days we were told to go and we went! The doctor visited the next day and gave me more information about what to expect, but I didn't care because I wanted something different. I returned to St. Anthony and a week later flew to Forteau. When I walked into the nursing station that first day, there were religious plaques everywhere, which made me nervous. Apparently that's what Sir Wilfred Grenfell wanted. There was pressure for me to go to a particular faith, and I was expected to do a Bible reading for the group each day, but I felt odd and kept saying I couldn't! Because I was a different colour they weren't sure what I was. On my vacation I bought a statue of a Hindu god and put it in my room and was never bothered again.

"When I started with Grenfell I took home $300 after my board and lodging at the nursing station and taxes were removed. Our salary came from the IGA office in Ottawa because we didn't have a finance office in St. Anthony until 1980 when the Government of Newfoundland took over responsibility for IGA.

"I got a good reception from the nurses on the coast. They liked it when somebody new came to tell them what was happening in England. They were also very supportive. I found St. Anthony very different from the Labrador coast, but they were used to people coming and going.

"Just as I arrived in Forteau I was told to go to Red Bay with the public health nurse. There was no such thing as an orientation! I changed into a white uniform, but it was a dirt road, so when I got there I was a brown nurse in brown clothes. There were 60 people in the clinic and the staff said, 'Everybody wants to see the new nurse so clinic will be busy.' The patients weren't expecting an Indian nurse and just stared. They said I had to treat the people and give medications. I was horrified! All I could think was, 'What if something happened?' Then part of me said, 'This is what you came for.' I could decide what was wrong and how to treat it, but I was petrified to give a prescription. I kept asking the doctor to come to the clinic to see if I was doing the right thing. He was amused but double-checked everything. The patients were irritated and amused. I could hear them through the wall saying, 'This new one isn't as good as so-and-so. She keeps you waiting some long!' The more I heard that, the more nervous I got!

"We finished at 10:00 p.m. and did three home visits on our way back. When we got back I discovered I was on call that night. I hadn't seen my room or unpacked my bags and the charge nurse's room was on the same floor, so I stayed downstairs on the couch. I didn't know what to do but staff told me when the patients' drugs were due. I was exhausted the next morning, but I wasn't going to show this British nurse I couldn't cut it. I knew the first day I made a mistake because these people needed more than I could give them. A personal care attendant said, 'You foreigners do what you like and nobody knows whether you are looking after our people or not.' I said, 'I'm scared, I just don't show it to patients.' But I did think, 'What have I done? Is it going to be like this every day?'

"I pulled teeth in Forteau and did things I'd never done before. The nurse came down when I did clinic and that's how I learned. We constantly debated treatments and drugs and whether to hold patients until a doctor visited, which was every six months. We were on our own except in emergencies. We discussed cases with a doctor on the RT where I'd give the history; he'd ask questions and make suggestions about what to do. They'd call one nursing station and while waiting their turn, all the others could hear everything. The head nurse left Forteau and they sent me somebody else because I didn't want to be in charge. I worked very independently, but when I look back it was the grace of God and common sense that made me calm in emergencies. I don't know how many times I said, 'These people need a doctor!'

"People in Forteau defrosted sewage pipes by lighting a fire in a drum. One day a drum exploded and hit the man in the skull. Somebody called to say they saw a truck racing from L'Anse aux Mort to Forteau and that 'He's hurt his head.' That's how they communicated messages! They parked the truck in front of the station; one nurse jumped in one end and I jumped in the other. We moved him into the hospital van and tried to put in an IV, but we knew he was dead. We just didn't tell the crowd. In Forteau everybody knows everybody, so it made sense to get out of the situation and we took him to Blanc Sablon hospital.

"We got a call from Capstan Island to come because someone had been shot. In those days our equipment was an IV and an oxygen tank. We jumped in the van with what we had, and an LPN and the maintenance man came with me. Normally it took 45 minutes to get there, but we did it in 15. The man had been shot in the chest. The bullet hole was tiny but the mattress was full of blood. I got an IV in but the man was dying. I called the doctor and she said to make him comfortable. We were hardly in the door when he died. The whole community was in the house, so I told the man's sister to have everybody leave and not touch anything. A young RCMP officer came and we put the body on the transport. The officer asked me to give the man's wife something because she was screaming and he was so worried about her. This was new for him also. He asked us to clean everything so the wife could return to the house.

"The wife said the four-year-old twins were playing with a gun and shot him, but everybody in the community said the wife shot him. I decided to go directly to Blanc Sablon, hand over the body, and do our report. Then we went back to Forteau and everyone wrote up what they saw because I knew this was going to be a problem. There was a murder inquiry and the RCMP officer had a disciplinary hearing. He wrote me later that he decided not to do police work again. I had another man die from a gunshot injury while thawing his gun over the stove.

"I had no work expectations when I went to the coast. I was told to work and I did. We worked 24 hours, six or six and half days a week, and rarely got a day off. Then the Public Health nurse said I should get two days off a week and should tell the nurse-in-charge that it was my right. She was absolutely floored and asked, 'When are we going to take two days off? There's no time.' And to be honest, there was no time. We had 2,500 people from L'Anse aux Clair to Red Bay with only two nurses. I said I'd like one Saturday off because everybody prayed on Sunday and nobody would take me Ski-Dooing or fishing. When I could, I got a half-day, and every so often I got a Saturday but rarely got two days off. If I was on-call at night I worked the next day because the work had to be done.

"I stayed in Forteau for two years then St. Anthony asked me to do the outpost nursing program. After I finished they asked me to go back to Forteau and I said, 'Yes,' if I could make changes. They sent me an English nurse and we made quite a few changes. We ordered up-to-date supplies because the older nurses had a missionary spirit and used groceries and supplies very judiciously, but those who came in the '70s had a very different perspective.

"They asked me to move from Forteau, but I said no. Usually if they wanted you to go to another nursing station, they picked up the phone and said, 'Pack your bags, you're leaving today.' They gave me six weeks off. I hadn't had a vacation because they'd say, 'You can go if we find another nurse.' You always booked a full-fare ticket because you never knew if they would change your vacation. I went across Canada with no intention of returning to Grenfell, but I got a call saying I could have a public health job in Cartwright or go to Nain. I went to Cartwright as the public health nurse for a year. The acute care nurse had been there for eight years and was delighted because she started to get days off. I'd do my home visits, then see what she wanted me to do and Grenfell was okay with that.

"I was asked to assist the Director of Community Medicine in North West River. I was nervous because the coastal nurses were a law unto themselves, but they were pleased a station nurse had been chosen.

These nurses were Trojans because some had no water, sewage that didn't work, and only surface water to bathe in. I thought that was appalling for this country. I gained credibility with them fairly quickly because I rolled up my sleeves to help and I tried to get things up to scratch in the stations. The station nurses were strong because they were advocates and made things work for their communities and had the community's respect. One nurse in Forteau managed to get the council to abolish drinking and there were no more liquor stores in the community. They were strong women, but I don't think St. John's recognized what they did up north.

"In 1990, I became Assistant Executive Director and was in that position for seven years until I became Interim Executive Director. It wasn't a job I wanted but I stayed for 16 months until I retired after 26 years and moved to St. John's.

"For a nurse who came from Kenya with no intention of staying, I stayed. The pull was Labrador, my friends, and family. I've stayed in this country longer than my own. I'm beginning to hate the snow in St. John's, but as you get older your support systems are here. There is no place to go. This is home."

❋

Aruna Thampy was born in Nairobi, Kenya. She graduated in 1970 as a KRN (Kenyan Registered Nurse) from Aga Khan Platinum Jubilee Hospital in Nairobi. In 1972 she completed midwifery as a SCM in England. Prior to immigrating to St. Anthony in 1975, she completed a neonatal course in Cornwall and an accident/emergency course in Liverpool.

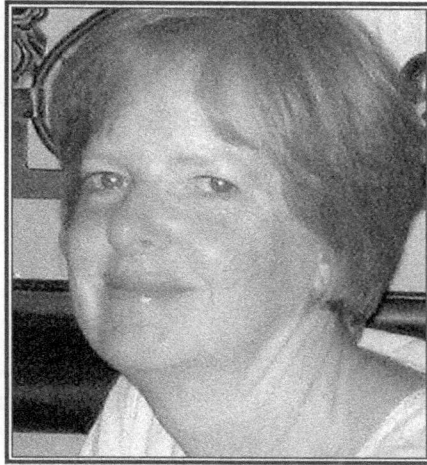

KARENE TWEEDIE

❊

1979

*"In some ways I feel very privileged to have had the career
I've had in Newfoundland. I've been happier in my career here than I
would have been elsewhere. Standards here are high."*

"I know this sounds corny, but the Scots are great travellers and I always wanted to travel. I was fascinated with Canada, particularly Newfoundland, because I learned about it in geography. Also I did a high school project on native peoples in the Arctic and was interested in the Inuit. I read a book about the Grenfell Association which attracted me, that romantic idea of what it might be like. I was about 16 or 17 when I originally wanted to come to Labrador or St. Anthony to do volunteer work. Now that was romantic because I didn't have a clue! I had no professional background so they said to re-apply when I had some qualifications, and after a lot of years I did. My brother came to Newfoundland first but he was qualified. I visited him in Grand Falls one summer and again in the winter and decided I would love to live here. Also I found it claustrophobic at home because you queued for everything, and it was so busy I thought, 'I want out. I want space and adventure.'

"I applied to the IGA's office in London. They sent information and I went there for an interview. Meanwhile I met a girl in Edinburgh who was also interested in going to Labrador. We read what we could and talked to people who had been there and got ourselves psyched up, but she met someone and didn't come. After I accepted a position I got a list of things to do, like get a work permit and contact ARNNL. Getting registered with ARNNL was probably the most frustrating part about the process. They had requirements, like eight weeks of OBS. My nursing program had four weeks and I had a hard job getting across that, as a midwife, I had more than eight weeks' obstetrics. That was a major challenge because we went back and forth about it. I wondered if it was worth it because that was a trial. I didn't have to write the Canadian RN exams because whoever came by 1979 was okay. I wrote them later because I was going to Nova Scotia and needed them to work in another province.

"I went to St. Anthony on a one-year work permit, although I almost didn't come. They wrote saying I'd be working in North West River. I talked to people who had worked there and was geared up to come. Two weeks before I left Scotland I got a letter from HR saying I was going to St. Anthony instead because that's where I was needed. I was very upset but then thought, 'I'll try it.' I could have transferred to North West River any time but I never did.

"I flew to Gander but the weather was down in St. Anthony, so I spent a week with my brother in Grand Falls. I got a phone call from HR saying, 'We're sending a plane tomorrow; be on it.' I got the plane to Deer Lake, then a driver from St. Anthony picked up me and another individual, and we drove up the Northern Peninsula, which was about 90 to 100 miles of dirt road. That was early February so it was late when we arrived. The driver took me to a nice house where I was to live with a bunch of other employees. I remember getting out of the van and standing there. The harbour was frozen, everything was snowy, and the stars were out. It was a beautiful night and so still, and I thought, 'I'm going to be here for a year.' I'd only met the driver and the other woman, but my first impression of the Northern Peninsula and St. Anthony was that I loved it. It may sound corny but I thought it was beautiful and exciting.

"I was introduced to the others in the house and they were great. There was a major party in full swing and everyone was half drunk and very friendly. I thought, 'This is wonderful, a great social life.' The person in London painted a false picture of what it was like because she said, 'Take a nice dress because you might go out one or two evenings, and take lots of books because there's not much to do.' My brother and sister-in-law phoned that night and said, 'How are you? What's it like? Are you lonely?' I had to say, 'I can't talk, we're having a party.' At that point I didn't have any regrets about coming.

"Grenfell paid my return airfare if I fulfilled a one-year term. Our accommodations were subsidized and we paid about $40.00. Ours was a big, old, lovely house with a nice garden. Four or five of us stayed there and I loved it. St. Anthony had a co-op and we went there, but often there were no bread or fresh vegetables because the trucks hadn't arrived. There were major transport problems in those days, so we ordered our groceries from the hospital kitchen. We'd get a list and tick off hamburger meat, milk, cornflakes, or whatever, and in a week or two we picked it up. We were limited in what we could get but the prices weren't as much as in the supermarket.

"I went to work the next day because I'd been in Grand Falls a week and had been on the payroll, so the hospital wanted me as quickly as possible. They told me I was going to psychiatry although I wasn't clear why. I said I was a midwife but they said my position was there. That was new to me, and had I known I wouldn't have come. I was on psychiatry three weeks but miraculously got on the obstetrical floor and worked there three years.

"I maybe got a couple of days orientation but my memory of it is vague. I was introduced to a supervisor who took me around the hospital and introduced me to everybody, and I was shown the policy and procedure manual. I probably had a few days' orientation to psychiatry but that's a blur. You learned on the job and went with another nurse to do things like meds. I didn't know much about the ARNNL then nor that I was in a union because some people frowned on it. We were kept away from that and I didn't learn about it until I left. People talked about the nursing strike of '79 but we didn't know anything about it. Several in management had a missionary view of work, but I never did. There was a balance between the missionary and regular types that somehow made work enjoyable.

"I was overwhelmed by how friendly everybody was. Before I got around the hospital during orientation I had several invitations to dinner. I wasn't used to such a welcoming atmosphere. A lot of staff came from the community and made their own fun. I had friends from Grenfell and friends who were local and everybody got on well. It was a good blend. I adapted easily because people were so friendly, generous and welcoming. They didn't lock their doors and would say, 'I won't be there but go into the apartment and make a cup of tea.' That was unusual for me, but I found it wonderful.

"Learning the language was very difficult because of the different terminology in nursing and for everyday things. In psychiatry I would be talking to people who were depressed, with their heads down, not making eye contact and mumbling. I was no use to them because I couldn't understand what they were saying.

"The majority of nurses and the head nurses in maternity at

St. Anthony were midwives so we were on the same wavelength. We worked the same as we did in the UK and maybe did things we shouldn't have. The forms were different but we didn't know the difference. As midwives we were limited because we needed an order for drugs like Demerol and we weren't used to that. Somebody would say, 'You need a doctor's order for that,' so we learned from those who had been here a while. We got an orientation about narcotics and double signing, but in retrospect many of us came from Britain or wherever and didn't know the difference, so we sometimes just did our own thing. As midwives we were in a privileged situation and maybe got to do things that others didn't.

"We had 23 antenatal and postnatal women, the nursery and labour area. We worked as a team where somebody did meds, somebody did dressings and somebody looked after the antenatal women or the postnatal women. Sometimes there was only one midwife for all areas, who could be in labour and delivery with somebody, so you depended on the nursing assistant to tell you if a patient needed something for pain or if an IV ran dry. Everybody worked together and the nursing assistants were excellent and kept us on track. We respected them and they respected us.

"In St. Anthony midwives didn't do deliveries outside the hospital unless we did a medevac for a maternity case. Even though I worked in maternity, I was still expected to go on medevacs, although that was always a grey area. They asked volunteers to go on their day off, but you didn't get paid. I'd go because I thought it was a wonderful adventure and a great opportunity. Later the union said we should get paid and couldn't work so many hours after doing a medevac. Unfortunately, somebody kicked up about getting paid, so we weren't asked to go much after that. I liked to go, although sometimes it was a bit hairy. I went on one by myself with an incubator to get somebody in premature labour. You'd have the drugs in your pocket and think, 'What am I going to?' We got there but the woman wasn't in premature labour. She wasn't even bleeding as badly as we were led to believe. I found the things you thought might be difficult weren't as bad when you got there. Then other times you went thinking it was something simple only to find much more than you bargained for.

"After St. Anthony I went to Corner Brook because it was time for me to move. I wanted somewhere bigger than St. Anthony but not St. John's. It was a whole different experience. My first day at the Corner Brook hospital was completely different from my first day in St. Anthony. I didn't get the same positive vibes. The people in Corner Brook weren't as friendly and there weren't as many people from the UK. I didn't enjoy my time in Corner Brook, and had I gone there first I would have gone home and never come back. Initially I worked on medicine and felt out of my league but thought it would be a challenge. Then I went to the case room as an obstetric nurse but found it a strain and frustrating. The nurses on the medical floor weren't welcoming, but the nurses in the case room were nice. I realized then that if I was staying in Newfoundland, I couldn't work as an obstetric nurse. I either had to go back to St. Anthony or Goose Bay or do something else. I went to MUN to do my BN and community health nursing.

"I sabotaged my midwifery career as soon as I left Scotland. I thought midwifery would be legislated here and did my master's in midwifery thinking it would happen. But I'll be finished my career before that happens! I live in Newfoundland because of the people. I'm not sure when I realized I was staying but probably when I started teaching at the Grace. I loved the people I worked with and enjoyed the work because by then I knew the ropes and the system. It was important to stay with people and a quality of life I like rather than pursue a midwifery career somewhere where I might not be as happy. I couldn't imagine going somewhere else.

"My family was always supportive, but I talked about coming here since I was a teenager. They would have thought I was crazy not to come. My parents have been here many times and never asked why I stayed. It might have been different if I'd been in Australia and my brother in Canada. They always encouraged us to do what we wanted. I know it was hard for them, because I overheard them talking and realized there were times when they wished we were around and missed seeing us. I go back and forth usually in the summer and at Christmas because my dad lives alone and his children are here.

"I would like to retire in Scotland but I can't see leaving here. It's a hard decision because I'm nearing the time when I have to think about it. I've spent more time here than in Scotland, and I don't know the system there now and find some things over there very frustrating. I'm more comfortable here in many respects because I have friends and a lot of ties. I would like the best of both worlds, a house in both places, but I'd need a lot of money to do that and somebody to look after them.

"The ideal would be to spend so many months in Scotland and so many months here. It's difficult to break links with your birth country, but I can't imagine leaving here after so long. When I came first I thought I'd died and gone to heaven because my salary was more than twice what I earned at home and the cost of living was much lower than at home. Financially I was a lot better off and could afford a much better lifestyle here. Even though the cost of living has gone up here, it is still higher at home. Life here is a lot easier, less stressful and a slower pace, and I love the open spaces. Also the working situation is more relaxed and less hierarchical. Nurses here have more rights and more say in their working conditions. In Scotland, nurses were expected to do what the supervisor told them and you didn't question. You took your orders! Here we are definitely treated better and are respected. In some ways I feel very privileged to have had the career I've had in Newfoundland. I've been happier in my career here than I would have been elsewhere. Standards here are high."

✳

Karene Tweedie was born in Edinburgh, Scotland, and graduated in 1977 as a Registered General Nurse (RGN) from Stobhill Hospital School of Nursing in Glasgow (two-year fast-track program following BSc in social sciences). She completed midwifery as a SCM at Simpson's Memorial Maternity Pavilion, Edinburgh, in 1978. She immigrated to St. Anthony in 1979.

STAN BURNS

☙

1981

[The immigration officer] ... asked if we knew where
we were going in Canada. I said, 'To Newfoundland.'
He took a deep breath and said, 'I repeat, you can go anywhere in
Canada.' I said, 'Well, boy, that's Newfoundland.'

"When we first came here my wife and I were just married. We planned to go abroad because we thought two nurses wouldn't get anywhere in the UK. I had jobs in Australia but my wife reneged because it was so far away and she couldn't stand the 24 hours to fly there and back. I saw a nursing magazine talking about the IGA in northern Newfoundland and Labrador. I wrote to someone in London and to ARNNL and found out we could register. I forgot to tell my wife what I had done! One morning she said, 'Have you got us jobs in Newfoundland?' I told her I applied, and she said, 'That was them on the telephone. We can go as soon as we get organized. I only have one question, where is it?'

"IGA sent the work visa application to complete and send to the Canadian Embassy and told the embassy we had positions in St. Anthony. ARNNL sent forms to complete, then notified us what was required when we arrived. Initially we both got temporary licences and I worked on that for a couple of weeks. My wife had to write the Canadian

RN exams for a permanent licence and had to wait six months for the next scheduled exams. I was exempt because I did obstetrics and ARNNL recognized the certificate. We came on a return commitment, which meant if we stayed two years they would fly us home. They didn't offer us anything else, although the salary was better than in England at the time, as was the exchange rate.

"I knew about Newfoundland because my mother remembered Newfoundland soldiers during the war. She knew where it was and was able to verse on it. She described them as characters, a bit like us, and I thought, 'If I'm going to move, go somewhere where they're like you and not too unfamiliar.'

"We came on a work visa for one year and extended for another year, but we were offered immigration right off the bat. Immigration called us into the office and said I completed the wrong papers. I said I filled out what they sent. But there wasn't a problem; they asked if we wanted to immigrate to Canada, not Newfoundland. I said it was a trial because we didn't know how we'd settle. What struck me was that she said, 'If you immigrate, you don't have to go to Newfoundland.' I thought, 'That's not very nice, what's wrong with Newfoundland?' We stuck to our guns and said, 'These people are paying to bring us over and we're going.' When we arrived there was a storm and we were in Gander for four days. IGA said to make ourselves at home and they would send the plane as soon as they could. They paid for hotels and everything. In Gander, people asked where we were going and when we said St. Anthony, they'd say, 'You need to get food in for the winter because you won't get anything by road.' My wife thought we'd have to eat at the hospital.

"My first impression of St. Anthony was 'Oh my God!' because there was nothing between the airport and the town. As we came into St. Anthony the first thing we saw was a fire station and as we moved through town I thought, 'This isn't bad. Quite a few people live here.' They drove us to our accommodations, which was a two-bedroom flat. In comparison to our accommodations in the UK this was paradise. There was central heating and in England we only had a fireplace in our sitting room. I thought, 'This is luxurious.' The fridge was stacked with eggs, milk, bacon and steaks. There was enough food for a week. They were well prepared for us.

"We got to St. Anthony on Friday and reported for work on Monday. We weren't given a lot of time to adjust, but sometimes that's better than having time to wonder about things. We got a short orientation: a couple of days explaining differences in practice and a couple of days on the floor. We also did CPR, which they don't tend to teach in the UK. I went to work in ICU immediately and after a few weeks when the charge nurse felt I was capable, I went in charge. But I didn't get an extended orientation before going in charge.

"The nurses at the hospital were excellent but they were used to British nurses. When we came, maybe 25 percent of the work force was from the UK, so we worked with people from a similar background to ours, which made it easy to settle in. There were some differences in nursing practice but nothing huge. But in those days Newfoundland nurses were mostly diploma-trained and had a lot of clinical background.

"I don't think you could meet nicer people in the world than the people in the community. They were very kind and generous and only too glad to help you, especially in your work. People just accepted you. I didn't have any major adjustments to life or the culture here, but I did have a few. I learned very quickly not to walk to the store in winter with only a little jacket and jeans on. I had to get a taxi back! I didn't realize how cold it was here, and I don't recall it being that cold in Scotland. I believe the culture here and in the British Isles, particularly Scotland, are similar, particularly the humour. My wife is from Waverley, a posh area of England, and it was probably more a shock for her than for me.

"I came from a large university hospital with 1,200 beds, 4,000 nurses, and 4,000 students. Sometimes we were staffed up to our ying-yang because there were a lot of students on the floor. I thought the nurses in St. Anthony worked harder than nurses in the UK. I never worked 12-hour shifts before, so they were foreign to me. After eight hours I was ready to go home. I got used to them but found I had too much time on my hands because I didn't need seven days off every two weeks.

"We went back to England in '83 because we were on work permits and my wife was pregnant. Also there were a lot of unemployed nurses in Ontario and some moved to the province. Nurses who had been here nine, ten years and thought their lives were here were told by immigration that their work permits were not being renewed, so they had to leave St. Anthony. Many planned to apply for immigrant status but didn't because they were told not to worry about it. Then suddenly the plug was pulled and they were sent home. In our case they had to advertise our jobs and if someone came forward with the qualifications we didn't get them. Fortunately nobody did and we kept our jobs. We went back to England and had a couple of kids. I had a good job with the Civil Service there, but we weren't getting anywhere fast because I was the only one working. Also we lived in the south of England where house prices are just extortionate. My salary wasn't bad but we still couldn't afford a house. One day my wife said, 'You're not very happy are you? Do you want to go back to Canada?' I said, 'I'd love to.' And I did, because here we had lots of friends and were always doing something. Also it was an opportunity to travel. I called the Canadian Embassy who sent the papers. We contacted people in St. Anthony who said if we came back they'd sponsor us. I reneged on that, though, because I didn't want to pay back time and I wasn't sure what we'd do or where we'd go. I wanted to come to St. Anthony because we knew the people and what was here, and I didn't want to start somewhere else. Also the houses were affordable. We had a good lifestyle here and enjoyed our work. So we decided to come back and take things from there.

"This time we had a different person at immigration in London. When we went into the office, the immigration officer told my wife to shut up because she wasn't the principal applicant and if I was allowed to immigrate she could come along. This is how we were spoken to! While I answered his questions, he wrote on a piece of paper because they tally your points and if you had sufficient points, you could immigrate. He said we had sufficient points and asked if I understood we could choose any port of entry into Canada. Then he asked if we knew where we were going in Canada. I said, 'To Newfoundland.' He took a deep breath and said, 'I repeat, you can go anywhere in Canada.' I said, 'Well, boy, that's Newfoundland.' It was fortunate I'd been here before, because that attitude would put people off if they wanted to come to Newfoundland and were relatively green.

"We stayed in St. Anthony seven months then moved to Gander for family lifestyle. We had two small children and my wife is also a nurse so babysitting was a problem. Our babysitters worked in the fish plant and when they were recalled to work they weren't available to us. Gander had preschools and nursery schools so we decided to come here. I will likely retire in Newfoundland, but I'm not sure it will be Gander. My sons are Newfoundlanders because my oldest boy was about three and my youngest boy just over a year when we came back, so their roots are here. One is in the Canadian military and the other is an electrician in St. John's. My roots are here as well, and I don't see my roots in the UK."

❧

Stan Burns was born in Glasgow, Scotland, and graduated in 1977 as a SRN in general nursing from South Hampton University Hospital, England. He completed neuromedicine and neurosurgery from the Joint Board of Clinical Nursing Studies and a diploma course in obstetrics from the UK Midwifery Council before immigrating to St. Anthony in 1987.

Chapter Six

St. Anthony Midwives

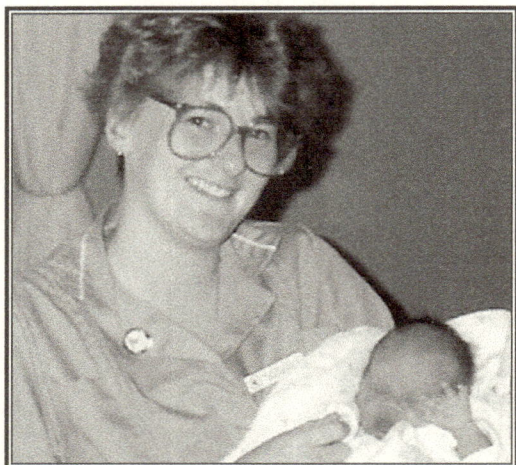

ALISON CRAIGEN

❋

1990

"The people in the community were friendly. It's a small place and everyone knows everyone else's business ... As soon as they see you, they'll say, 'That must be the new midwife,' because everyone knows there's a new midwife coming."

"Seventeen years ago I came from Edinburgh, Scotland, for one year. I came over in response to the need for midwives and fancied going somewhere, so I applied for two jobs advertised in the *Midwifery Chronicle*: one in New Zealand and one here. I heard from New Zealand first and my mother was desperate for me to go because she's got family there. But it was too far away and Grenfell really sells themselves. They make it sound so exciting with polar bears and icebergs. St. Anthony was closer to home, but the biggest plus was that Grenfell paid my way out and I had to pay my airfare to New Zealand. Much to my mother's dismay I came here.

"I came to St. John's on Friday and had a real problem because I couldn't understand what they were saying. I didn't think I was in Canada, I thought I had landed in Ireland! I cried almost the whole way over and thought, 'What the hell am I doing?' I had to phone the hospital in St. Anthony and couldn't get it to work. A man offered to help me but I couldn't understand a word he was saying. I spent the night in St. John's and was fascinated with the big trucks and fancy cars, because in the UK everyone has little cars. It was just like you'd see on TV. I got a taxi to the hotel and the driver must have thought, 'This one is crazy!' The traffic lights were suspended in the middle of the road and I kept saying, 'Look at the traffic lights! Look at the trucks! Wow, look at the cars!'

"I flew to St. Anthony on the hospital plane on Saturday, and flying in I thought I was in God's country. It was a nice day in St. John's but St. Anthony was wet and overcast and I thought, 'Where am I going?' When I arrived, RT gave me a key and a security guard took me to the apartment I was sharing with two other girls. Someone was supposed to meet me but nobody was there. Then on Monday I got a gift basket. I unpacked my suitcase and lay on the bed, crying. I think you're in shock that you've actually made the move. There was a group of us and we got a couple of weeks' orientation about Grenfell's policies and procedures, CPR, and fire drill, then they showed us around the hospital. I also got a couple of weeks' orientation to the ward.

"I only planned to stay for one year and was dreadfully homesick. In December I went to Boston with a girl I had met here. My mom and dad met us and my mom kept saying, 'You're coming home when the year's up, aren't you? Promise you'll come home. You've not met anybody have you?' I said, 'I'll come home.' Then two days after I got back here I met my future husband. It was first time we met and also my birthday. He bought me a gift and I thought it was very romantic. We got engaged in February and were married in June. My husband is from Cook's Harbour. It's about a half hour from St. Anthony and has a population of about 200 people. We were married here and they were all at our wedding. I knew maybe 50 people at my wedding; the others were total strangers. I wanted my family to come but it was too much money. But we got married in Britain that October, so we did it twice!

"Nursing was pretty much the same here as home, although there were different names for medications and IV solutions. I had difficulty understanding patients because I had trouble with the accent. Sometimes I'd say, 'What did you say?' or get someone to tell me what the patient was saying. But the patients were good and they'd say, 'That's the way we talk!' Seventeen years later the patients are still polite and will repeat things if I'm having trouble. But the language differences resulted in a funny story. One of my nursing friends slept in one day and was late for work. The security guard went to wake her and when I asked how she got up, she said, 'The security guard knocked me up.' Of course everyone laughed at that and her father-in-law thought it hilarious that the security guard was going around knocking up the women in morning! When I would get petrol they'd say, 'It's not petrol, it's gas!' My husband told me to ask for tin foil and when I asked for aluminum foil, they got a kick out of that. Here a housecoat is a duster, but to me a duster is a rag you clean with. Things like that were different.

"The nurses were friendly but there was a problem with my accent and theirs and understanding what we were each saying. But the head nurse on the ward was also a Scots woman who had been here for 20 years. St. Anthony is a small place and everyone knows everyone else's business, which can be a bit of a nuisance, but it really doesn't matter. As soon as they see you, they'll say, 'That must be the new midwife' because everyone knows there's a new midwife coming. But everyone here is very friendly.

"I work on OBS at the hospital, although we also have pediatrics, general surgery and medicine. If they're busy elsewhere I have to help out as an RN. Midwives do normal deliveries, but if a woman in labour needs a caesarian section we go to the OR with them because we do the nursing. And when somebody is in labour we're with them, but we do nursing if there's no one in labour and delivery. Comparing OBS to the UK, women here are much stronger. They don't require pain relief like they do in the UK, but the reason for that is the ladies here get to know us because they live in the area or they come from Labrador for scans. It's a much nicer relationship. I delivered the third baby of the woman who was my first delivery when I came. I delivered all three of the children of our physiotherapist. I wasn't working for her third and it was five in the morning, but she refused to push until they phoned me and I delivered the baby. People stop me in the drugstore and tell me they're pregnant and it's really lovely when people come up to you. People here are so much friendlier and you miss that in a big city.

"My mom has been to St. Anthony but she hates it because she loves big city life and shopping. This is so far away and there are no shops so she doesn't come very often. Also she's 72 now so travelling is harder. My father, on the other hand, loves it here. He was here for a month in July and is coming next month for three months. If he could get organized he might retire here. I go to Scotland every couple of years. We went for my mom's 70th birthday and will go next year for my nephew's wedding. I would go back to Scotland but my father doesn't live there anymore. My mom wants me to come home so they can help with the kids, but I don't like where she lives.

"If my family were in Scotland I might move, but I'm 42 and the thought of packing to move and starting a new job!

"Nursing practice is the same, but it means getting into a new system and I'd just as soon stay here. Also my children are used to Newfoundland. My son has attention-deficit and is set up with his doctor and the school system. Not that it is the best, but he is a factor because in a bigger place he might get lost in the system. Also I have to feel safe and secure, and here my children have more freedom and I have less worry. I'm divorced but still call on my mother-in-law because she'll always be my mother-in-law. Her family is very good and the children spend a lot of time with them. They help out with child-care but my family would also. I've worked since I came here and have 17 years invested in a pension, and I'm looking into whether I can claim my UK pension. Chances are that I am not going back to my family now. Canada is home for my kids."

❋

Alison Craigen was born in Elgin, Scotland, and graduated as a SRN from Worthing Health Authority in Sussex, England, in 1986. She completed midwifery as a SCM from Simpson's Memorial Maternity Pavilion Hospital in Scotland in 1989 and immigrated in 1990 to work as a midwife at the hospital in St. Anthony.

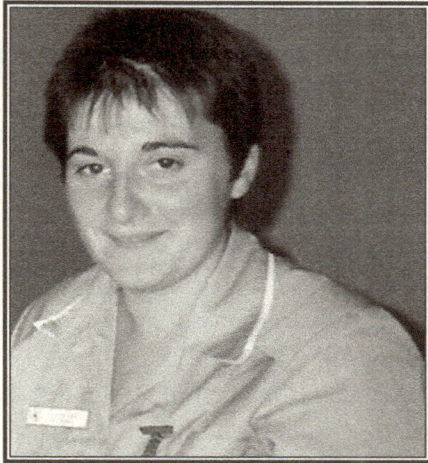

GILLIAN (SAGE) SEXTON

※

1990

*"Grenfell ... doesn't realize that in England you don't know
what wilderness is ... I'd never seen wilderness. England has fields ...
but there are not hundreds of miles of nothing. I'd never experienced
winter and when I came in April the sea was frozen!"*

"I planned a vacation to volunteer overseas, but a nun said, 'Perhaps you
should try living in an English-speaking country abroad before you go
to the third world and see how you manage in a developed country that's
away from home.' It was a voluntary thing and you had to commit for
two years and stay wherever you were posted unless you got sick. There
were two advertisements in a midwifery journal: one for here and one for
New Zealand. I put my application in for both places and IGA called me

within a month and asked, 'Can you come tomorrow because we're desperate?' From that call until I arrived here was six months. They called in October and I started the paperwork in December. I faxed my resume and they checked my references. I was naïve about the immigration process. I went up to Immigration in London and was in a queue for two hours! I did what I thought I had to do, but they called and said I needed another interview in London. When I said I lived in Bristol they must have called St. Anthony because they waived my interview, but I couldn't tell anybody. I came in through the back door but I had all the paperwork done.

"When I told everyone I was coming here, they said, 'What are you doing?' But I talked to a nurse who had worked here for a couple of years as a midwife and as a regional nurse and really enjoyed it. That made my decision to come much easier. Grenfell sends a very interesting package that says it's a rural area, but in England you don't know what wilderness is. I'd never seen wilderness. England has fields and is a little bit like here with the villages, but there are not hundreds of miles of nothing. I'd never experienced a winter and when I came in April the sea was frozen! I didn't realize how far north I was coming and a map doesn't do justice to the miles.

"Grenfell told me to book my ticket and I went to the local travel agent. I said I wanted to go to St. Anthony, Newfoundland, and we had to get the map to find it. They said it was in Canada but I thought it was in Ireland. I came to St. John's and Grenfell gave me a number to call and arrange transport to St. Anthony. I phoned the RT, who said, 'Go to the Hudson General.' I asked if it was the train station and the guy on the phone fell off the chair laughing because there are no trains in Newfoundland. The hospital plane came to pick me up and they were bringing in a psychiatric patient who was in a straitjacket. That was my first introduction to Grenfell! The nurse was from Australia and he said, 'Good day, you must be Gillian, the new midwife. We've been waiting for you for three months.' It was nice to come on the hospital plane because they were so used to welcoming new staff.

"In those days hospital security drove people back and forth to the airport by bus and RT organized the duties for welcoming new staff. Grenfell provided accommodation so you knew you had somewhere to live. We paid for it but at a reduced rate. When you arrived RT was expecting you and had the key to your apartment, and security took you there. I remember the security guard saying, 'You're living with [name] but she got sent on medevac.' We shared accommodations in those days so he took me up to mine, which was in the old Grenfell orphanage. I thought it was a room but it was an apartment with a living room, kitchen, three bedrooms, and a bathroom. He opened the fridge and said, 'Help yourself to food. [Name] won't mind.' I remember think-ing, 'I don't know this girl!' But she had left a note saying, 'Gone on medevac. There's milk, tea and coffee. Help yourself.' In England, you would never do that. I worked in an environment where everything was locked up. But here people just assume that everybody knows everybody.

"It was spring when I arrived but not like in England, because there was snow down. I dressed for what I thought was cold weather but it was freezing. They told me to wear boots but mine were dress boots. My mom said to take my winter coat, but it was 60 degrees Fahrenheit when I left England and my winter coat certainly wasn't warm enough for here. They also said to bring ski clothes because I might need them in the spring, and they did me for the spring but they wouldn't have done through the winter.

"There were no incentives to come except they paid your way out. If you stayed a year you didn't have to pay that money back, but when you went home you paid your way. Also, the wages were a bit higher than in England at the time. Grenfell paid for the immigration and offered to help you get landed immigrancy if you stayed. They paid for my landed immigrancy. Grenfell was good at recruiting people because they offered them something different.

"I arrived on Friday and went to work on Monday because the staff education people were off Saturdays and Sundays and they couldn't start my orientation earlier. IGA had such a big turnover of staff and everyone had their little quirks for doing stuff, so they gave you a week of general orientation for some continuity. When I went for orientation, I walked to the hospital. I didn't know where to go but I saw a door and headed that way. Within two minutes somebody said, 'Oh, you must be ....' I only got two days' orientation to the ward. The first morning I went there one of the girls said, 'Are you the new midwife? Go around the corner. They've had three deliveries and another one is pushing.' I didn't know where 'round the corner' was! I walked around and a girl was in a room with no equipment, and sure enough, she was pushing. I'm shouting, 'Help!' because I didn't know where the drugs or anything were.

"My initial impression of St. Anthony was that everything was different. Our apartment didn't have a phone, so it was difficult calling England until we got it hooked up a couple of days after I came. When I called home, Mom asked what it was like but I couldn't describe it. I kept saying, 'Well, it's white and there are wooden houses.' How do you describe something so different from home? I said it looked like a fishing village in Cornwall but without the steep cliffs. She wanted to know what I meant by wooden houses and I said, 'They're shaped like home but made of wood.' At the end I said I couldn't stay and she wanted to know why. When I said, 'They're not speaking English,' she said, 'Don't be so ridiculous.'

"But everyone talked so fast, especially people from Goose Cove where I live now. The only thing I understood was my name. It was the same with clients and mums. They spoke so fast and I'd listen but only get one word in three or four. They were so used to midwives that they assumed I was like everybody else even though I was new. They would say, 'I'm sick,' meaning they were in labour and I'd never heard the term. I remember my second delivery when this gentleman from Labrador kept calling all morning and asking, 'Is my wife sick?' I'd say, 'No, you're wife's fine; she's in labour.' This went on until lunch time when I told him on the phone that he had a son because husbands didn't come in in those days. He must have thought, 'This is a stunned one I got here. That's what I've been asking all day!'

"I didn't have difficulty adapting to the nursing practices although they were a bit different. Drugs were the big thing because the names were different and Canada uses different drugs from England so that took a while. Transcribing orders was a big headache because I wasn't used to that. In England we did rounds but there were no fixed doctor's orders to sign off every day. The nurse did the nursing. Here, a nurse does not have the same autonomy because the doctors control everything. I never heard of a doctor ordering vital signs or bowel sounds; we assessed bowel sounds even after bowel surgery. The nurse decided the patient's diet and if she wasn't sure, she called the dietician. I still find it strange to see some of the orders that are written, like 'mobilize somebody.' You know I'm going to walk them!

"When I first came the drugs were just archaic. We poured them in pots with names on a tray and then carried them around to give them out. A lot of the midwifery practices in St. Anthony were set up along English lines because the doctors at Grenfell trained in England and were used to midwives. That benefitted us and made things similar. When I first came, Grenfell didn't have as much equipment as I was used to. Most hospitals had pumps but we only had one or two in ICU. In England we had a computer system but here we didn't even have a computer. Here, we still handwrite the forms going to government whereas in England you pressed a button and the birth notice and discharge forms were automatically sent. In England things were becoming very litigation-based, especially in midwifery, so it was refreshing to come here where it wasn't like that and still isn't. That gave us a bit more freedom. I'm glad I'm a midwife because we practice outside of the nursing body. I write my own orders and discharge and admit people without a doctor's order.

"Another big problem in health care when I came was that Labrador had no roads, and here there were dirt roads so when you went on medevacs, you were on your own. You could call from the plane through the pilot, but relaying through the pilot was difficult.

"The nurses were very friendly when I came, but my first summer here they changed the staffing policy on OBS. They moved the LPNs to surgery and only RNs were going to be on obstetrics. There was resentment about that. A couple of years later, pediatrics closed and there was resentment then too. As midwives, we had one of the more secure jobs in the hospital because Newfoundlanders didn't have the qualifications to do the job. Also, at that time we had one obstetrician, three GPs, and 50 deliveries a month, so they needed midwives and we knew we weren't going to be displaced.

"As friendly as people were, when it came to job security, they didn't say anything to our face and they were never rude to us, but there was an undercurrent. I've been here so long now that I'm senior, but that time was difficult. I could understand their feelings, especially those who had invested money in coming back. Some had bought houses and were planning to settle in the area. And then there were the big changes like splitting the health care board, which caused umpteen bad feelings in the area because then you had the 'Labrador versus Northern Peninsula' thing. For a while we just kept our heads down and did our job. But by then a lot of the nurses were having babies and wanted a midwife, so there was a need for us.

"The community was really friendly when I came, but midwives have been part of this community forever, not only trained but also lay midwives. My husband's grandmother was a midwife so in his family it was very normal. I met him through a group of nurses who knew him from being around in St. Anthony. If someone was having a party you were invited to come along and within a few months you were doing the downtown thing. In no time you met people and they included you. The ward clerk invited three of us to dinner and she served figgy pudding for lunch. We said, 'Do we eat that with the meat?' because at home we'd have it with custard. Shortly after I got here I was in a long line in the bank and people in the line said, 'You must be one of the new midwives. We've been waiting for you.' Then somebody said my name and I thought, 'How do they know I'm the new midwife?' That would never happen in England. But I don't think they see us as foreign now because we're part of the environment and committed to the community. I volunteer in the community and people got to know us away from the hospital. It's different now.

"St. Anthony wasn't a foreign environment for me because the director of nursing was English and the staff was mainly foreign nurses. Newfoundland nurses didn't come back here to work, which amazed me, and I found that really strange. In many ways St. Anthony is very small, but the staffing at the hospital makes it very international. Children here are used to foreign children. It's not unusual for them to grow up with children who are black or don't speak English as their primary language. The children here are raised with that and love it. They think it's marvelous.

"My friend got married our first year here so I stayed for her wedding then went home. She came home to have her wedding blessed and I went to that too. I was working casual as an agency nurse, which meant I might have to travel 40 miles between hospitals around Bristol for an eight-hour shift. I was fed up working casual and also I didn't want to work in an English hospital where you did delivery for a while, then postnatal for a while. Work was a good thing for me, but I had lived in big cities where the hassle of going to and from work was sinful. Also I realized how crowded England is and I marvelled at it. My friend suggested I come for the winter, which I did, and that is how I met my husband and stayed. I had no difficulty getting back the second time. When I called they were in a shortage situation, which was usual. They asked if my work permit was still good and it was, so they said, 'Come on.' I came two weeks before Christmas. They paid my flight back again. But I also loved the work here where I do everything. I love the continuity, which fits midwifery, because here you follow a mom from start to finish and see the babies born. Then I come home ... after working a night shift, it's a beautiful day; in 10 minutes I'm home and what a view! In England I'd be in all the traffic.

"Another thing about coming here are the medevacs, which is a nice side of nursing and expands your experience. It can be frightening, like the day I took a patient to St. John's. She was 28 weeks with severe hypertension. It was before we had monitors or phone packs. All I had was a blood pressure cuff, which I couldn't use on the plane. Another time they asked me to go to Goose Bay hospital to pick up a child in a body cast and I ended up in Nain for a gunshot wound. All I had in the medevac bag was a couple of IV bags and I'd never been there before. I had the pilot put down in Goose Bay and I told them I wasn't qualified to go but I ended up going. It was winter and they brought the patient on a komatik across the ice to the plane and the doctor says, 'He's not very stable, who do you have with you?' I said, 'Me and an obstetric bag'—but we got him to Goose Bay fine.

"I was hired as a midwife but there are days when I'm not needed as a midwife. But that's another thing that attracts me here because I don't want to give up nursing duties either. I really like the midwifery and I enjoy the nursing. The work here is good. Grenfell also offered CPR and other courses free, whereas in England they were charging for them. I did a medevac course here, which would have been expensive at home. Also, Grenfell sponsored you to do courses even if you were only here a year. They invested money in your development. And if you wanted to work on the coast they were pretty accommodating in letting you go.

"My parents came for a holiday and I spent a few days with them in St. John's because if the hospital plane was going to St. John's and there was room you could put your name down to go. I flew back to St. Anthony because I was working and they hired a car. I told them that on the drive up, there was a hotel at Hawkes' Bay with a restaurant, another one at Plum Point, and then St. Anthony, so be at one of these for lunch. They got to Plum Point about 5:00 and because I was working until 8:00 p.m., they went into the restaurant. When the lady at the restaurant realized they were English, she said, 'You must be Gil's parents. Hold on, I've got something for her.' My father, who is very chatty, was absolutely silent for the rest of the meal. When he saw on the map that they were 150 miles from St. Anthony, he couldn't understand how they knew me. But the woman was one of my first deliveries and was sending me a baby picture. My mom said my father never got over it. I found that different too when I came. I lived in Bristol where there were 5,000 deliveries. Women came in, delivered, but I never knew them and never saw them again. Within a couple of months of coming here, I knew the women and saw the babies I delivered in the community.

"The first time my family met my husband, we went home for a holiday. They were frightened having this strange person in the house and Mom kept saying, 'What are we going to do for three weeks?' By the time we left, Mom said, 'I like him,' and that was when they realized I wasn't coming home anymore. It's been hard for Mom because she has two grandchildren she doesn't see. Once my parents retired it was easier because they bought a place here. They came for six weeks this summer and some years they might come three times. Mom would move here but dad doesn't like winters. He came one winter for my daughter's birthday in February and we had an ice storm with no electricity for three days. That put him off forever, but they love it here and can see the benefits of life here. People think my kids miss out on stuff, but they don't. So much goes on here for children and it's so much cheaper. Mine can go on the back path on their bikes and I'm not worried. They can be involved in things like hockey or skating, although there are things that are seasonal, like they can't swim all year long.

"I came for a year and it was like a well-paid working holiday where I worked full-time and got lots of experience. It was like living away from everything because you weren't involved in the work politics that is everywhere and you didn't have to worry about the longevity of things. I do miss being home for birthdays, anniversaries and weddings. I'm probably the first to know if someone in the family is getting married because if I get advance notice I can go home. But every now and then I do miss things because I've lost a couple of aunts and uncles and my grandmother, but I just can't always get home. I do go home every two years."

❋

Gillian (nee Sage) Sexton was born in Bristol, England, and graduated as a SRN in general nursing from the Royal Devon Exeter School of Nursing in 1986. She completed midwifery as a SCM in Taunton, Summerset, in 1987 before immigrating in 1990 to work as a midwife at the hospital in St. Anthony.

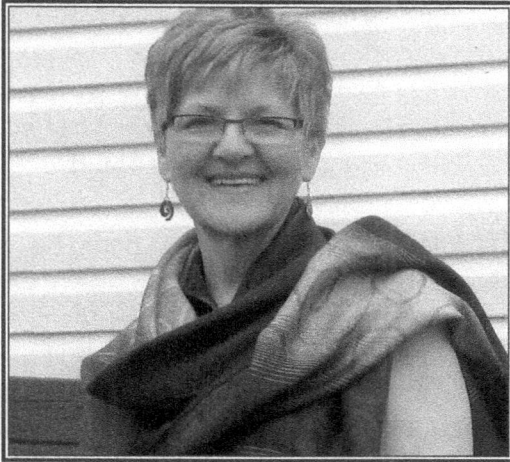

SYLVIA (JONES) PATEY

❋

1994

*"When people ask if I'm happy here I always say, 'I would rather
live in Newfoundland and visit England than live in England as
it is now and visit Newfoundland.' It just doesn't compare."*

"My mother was a war bride who married a Canadian, and I was told
that if I immigrated I had a birthright to Canadian citizenship one year
after I landed in Canada. I pursued immigration for 10 years but kept
hearing I didn't have the qualifications needed for employment in
Canada because I only had a nursing qualification. In 1991 I did
two years midwifery, qualified and worked as a midwife. I was still
pursuing immigration but kept coming up against a brick wall. I got so

frustrated that I phoned about my application and was told it had failed. I cried and said I wanted to speak to a supervisor. I was very assertive and the young man didn't know what to make of this blithering woman on the phone. He got the supervisor and I told her I had been trying to get to Canada for 10 years. She said I needed work and asked what I did for a living. I told her I was a midwife. She said to keep trying and that she would have the secretary of the Canadian Embassy call me. Meanwhile I saw an advertisement in a 1986 midwifery magazine for midwives for St. Anthony. I thought, 'No way will it still be there but I'm going to write anyway.' I wrote in August and got a phone call in October from the HR person in St. Anthony. He said, 'You applied for a job as a midwife and we'd like to offer you a position. We haven't one just now but expect to have one soon because we have a high turnover. We'll keep your application on file.' There I was, up one minute and down the next!

"The next day I phoned immigration in London, asked to speak to the Canadian Immigration Secretary and they put me through! She said, 'I am looking at your application and would like you to come to London for an interview.' I was very nervous when I went because there were a lot of multicultural people waiting but I didn't have to wait. This elegant Canadian woman told me she had read my file and would process my application. She said, 'I have a place in my heart for children of war brides.' She asked about my qualifications and I told her I had a promise of a job in St. Anthony, Newfoundland, as a midwife. She said, 'You'll love it there; it's like the west coast of Scotland.' At that point I had never heard of Newfoundland! Then she told me what had to be done. She skipped the police exam because I never had any crimes. She wanted to see my parents' marriage certificate and would process the rest.

"At Christmas I got a call from the guy in St. Anthony asking if I could come by January, and I told him I didn't know if I'd be processed in time. I contacted the lady at Canada House who said everything would be processed by the end of January. I flew to Canada in January 1993 and left my family behind. I had a terrible time getting to Canada because everything was snowed in. I was re-routed from Toronto to Montreal and was on my own. I came early to spend a week with my cousins in Ontario and had a very traumatic day realizing the enormity of what I'd done! My cousin said, 'Look at it this way, if you don't like it you can go back.' I thought that once I signed on the dotted line that was it.

"I arrived in St. Anthony the first week of February. When I landed at the airport I thought, 'What have I done?' The hospital bus picked me up and as we drove into St. Anthony I was excited and scared at the same time because all I saw was snow and ice, but then I saw the town and was thrilled. The driver took me to the hospital, got some keys, and then took me to Carlson House. I settled in for a weekend on my own because I didn't know a soul and didn't start work until Monday. It was a beautiful weekend so I walked around the community to buy a radio. The lady in the shop asked if I worked at the hospital and where I was staying. I showed her where I lived and she told me I could cut across what I thought was a field. I saw Ski-Doos zipping across that same field and I'd never seen them in my life. She told me to be careful of the Ski-Doos and just follow the tracks. She never told me it was the harbour! I didn't know until somebody at work told me and I freaked. I never walked on water before!

"Orientation was two weeks and I was fortunate to have an English educator which helped a lot. She said, 'Talk to the people in the community because sometimes the nurses and doctors who come to St. Anthony make the mistake of closeting themselves in their apartments after work and never mix with people in the community.' I'll never forget that because it was a wonderful tip and I met some marvelous people. This woman was married to a Newfoundlander and invited me to supper where I met her family. They invited me to eat many times after that and I met their friends. By the time I met patients on the ward I was somewhat familiar with the difference in language and the patients probably understood me better than I understood them. I was fortunate because I worked with English nurses and midwives who had been here many years. I remember one night running back to the desk to ask, 'What's a step-in?' That was the name used by ladies from the Straits for a pair of underwear. This lady wanted me to get a pair from her bag, but I didn't know if I was looking for pajama bottoms or what! The girls laughed! That was the beginning of many new words I learned. When I'd ask a patient, 'What is your main problem?' they'd say, 'I have a wonderful pain in my back,' and I'd think, 'A wonderful pain!' I kept a book of these things. When I came first I'd write home every day and put these wonderful sayings in. Another thing that startled me was the amazing names they gave their babies, like Ocean. Some names just blew me away, names we didn't hear in England. A lot of them came from the television stories.

"It took me about six months to adapt to the documentation and having to have a doctor's order for absolutely everything! In England we follow the nursing process just like here. We documented in the care plan, which was filed in the patients chart. We did ward rounds with the consultant and if he wanted an x-ray or something done, he wrote it in the patient's notes and we took it from there. We never rang a doctor to give a patient a glycerine suppository or Tylenol. They weren't prescribed. If we wanted to change a patient's diet, we changed it. I found that terribly frustrating here! When I left England any nursing care I did, I entered it into the patient's record on computer. We didn't write all these notes, although you did expand on some things as needed.

"I've had some wonderful experiences here as a midwife. The best one was the year I came. I did the medevac course in October, and in November was asked to go on a medevac to pick up a lady in William's Harbour, Labrador, which was not accessible by road and the nearest nursing station was Mary's Harbour, two hours away by boat. The plane picked me up and it was a beautiful, cold day and I was really excited! The woman was having abnormal vaginal bleeding, and I had to bring her back because the gynecologist obstetrician was in surgery at the time. We circled over William's Harbour, which was scary because they said they hadn't landed on the airstrip before. To me the runway looked like an aircraft carrier jutting out to sea. When they landed I was in the back of the plane with my eyes closed! We were picked up by a truck full of men. Our equipment was put in the truck and we were driven over a bumpy road into the community. When the driver told me that 77 people lived in the community I was so excited. When I walked into the house, all these men were sitting around the table drinking coffee and eating bakeapple cheesecake. Then I heard the familiar noise of a woman bearing down and one of the men said, 'She's up there nurse.' I went up and there were some women around the bedroom door looking in. There was also a nurse who was very flustered. She said, 'She's delivering,' and I said, 'I can tell.' I always took a delivery bag so I delivered the baby, which was 36 weeks gestation, and there were no problems. The woman got up, had a bath, we went downstairs and had lunch, then I flew back to St. Anthony. It was the most wonderful experience of my life and I realized I was so blessed because we weren't allowed to do home deliveries in St. Anthony.

"The requirement when I came was that I work as a nurse and a midwife at the hospital but I found it hard having to be both. In England you are either a nurse or a midwife. You're not one cap one minute and another cap the next. At nine in the morning here I could be bathing an old lady with a fractured hip or cleaning a colostomy, and then half an hour later I could be admitting a lady to the labour room and having to stay with her until she delivered. On nights we had only one nurse and a midwife on, and the midwives had to help on the floor. Midwives could relieve anywhere in the hospital but the nurses couldn't relieve us. Here we could be in the labour room for 12 hours without a break, whereas in England a team of midwives worked on a central delivery suite and when you took your break somebody relieved you, but you didn't leave the unit. Also midwifery was far more autonomous in England. Things here are very legalistic. I felt with documentation I was duplicating and duplicating and thought it was a waste of time. At home you entered any nursing care you did into the computer for the patient. It seemed here you spent more time doing paperwork instead of being with the patient.

"I planned to stay here a year and then move to Ontario. But then I bought a house and met my husband. I'm very happy I came to Newfoundland. I have experienced a lot of turmoil in my lifetime, and although I was born in England and spent 40 years there, I never felt at home or at peace there. Buying my first house in Newfoundland wasn't a hard decision. I remember sitting on the chesterfield looking out over the harbour because I'd always wanted to live by the water and the view out my window was my dream. I said, 'Sylvia, at last you're home,' and I felt at peace. It was a difficult decision to leave my family in England, and it is still heart-wrenching when I leave them to come back here. But when I come back to Newfoundland, I'm just as excited about coming home as I am going to England. When people ask me if I'm happy here I always say, 'I would rather live in Newfoundland and visit England than live in England as it is now and visit Newfoundland.' It just doesn't compare."

❋

Sylvia (nee Jones) Patey was born in Southhampton, England, and graduated as a SRN from Doncaster School of Nursing in Yorkshire, England. She completed midwifery as a SCM at the Royal Infirmary in Doncaster in 1991 and immigrated to St. Anthony to work as a midwife in the hospital in 1994.

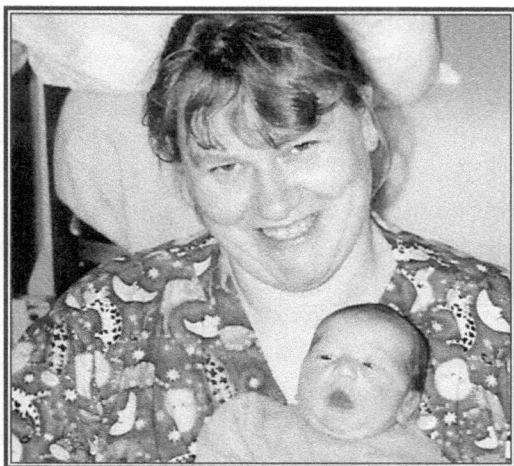

HELEN (WHEATLEY) PENNEY

❋

1997

*"I applied on a whim, they called and offered me the job and
that was it. They asked if I'd come for a year and I said, 'Yes,' although
I didn't know where it was or anything about it."*

"When I was in training I got the *Nursing Times* magazine and every
couple of years St. Anthony advertised for midwives and I liked the job
description. I always wanted to be a midwife but didn't want to stay in
the UK, so I thought, 'When I finish midwifery I might do that!' When
I qualified as a midwife the job never came up. I applied to the States
and was going to take the US exams when the job was advertised again.
I thought, 'I wouldn't mind doing that.' I applied on a whim, they

called and offered me the job and that was it. They asked if I'd come for a year and I said, 'Yes,' although I didn't know where it was or anything about it.

"I spoke to a manager here at the time who painted a very dreary picture of a little isolated community. I imagined it was a tiny community in the middle of nowhere, completely isolated from the rest of the world with little or no electricity, like the show *Northern Exposure*. I was picked up at the airport and as we drove into town I saw a shopping mall, electric lights and power lines. I was so excited! I thought I'd come to a big metropolis. She told me later that she painted that picture because so many people came with an idea in their head and no matter what she told them they were disappointed at how isolated it was when they got here. I sold everything in the UK, including my house, packed my furniture, and burned all my bridges. I arrived Halloween 1997 and lived in Carlson House, which was owned by the hospital and had one-bedroom apartments. My neighbour there was one of the midwives who met me, brought me to the hospital, and showed me around. I didn't know anybody but people were really friendly.

"Language was a big thing but there were lots of English nurses who helped me. On one of the first days I worked, a patient asked me to draw the machine around the bed. I looked for something mechanical but she kept saying, 'The machine, maid, the machine!' I'm thinking, 'What machine?' I didn't know what she wanted, but it was the curtain you pull around the bed.

"In the UK, midwives wore dress uniforms and where I worked in the labour room you could be squatting on the floor, hanging in the birthing pool, delivering on the floor or in all kinds of positions and your dress would be up around your waist! It was just so impractical, but here we wear scrubs which are much more practical. We don't have a birthing pool here and we don't do water births. Also in the UK, midwives do home deliveries but I was hospital-based, although I was involved in a couple of home deliveries. In England we worked eight-hour shifts but here it's 12-hour shifts. I like them and the days off are nice, but 12 hours is a long time to be away from your kids.

"Midwifery is the same as in England but here I am also employed as an RN. We work on the obstetrical floor but can get anything from pediatrics, orthopedics, mental health, female surgery, or medicine and geriatrics. Some of these areas were a challenge, especially pediatrics, because I hadn't done them since training. We do antenatal clinics, first visit clinics, and anything pertaining to midwifery and pregnant women, and if there's nothing in the labour room we work on the floors as RNs. If there are postnatal or antenatal women on the floor we look after them, but so do the RNs. We all work together and it's nice. It's busy here and we have been caught on the hop a couple of times.

"I was here three weeks when I got set up on a blind date with Robert, my husband, and we now have two children. I've been back to England a couple of times and Robert has been also. I'm not lonely here because everybody's really friendly and Robert's family is excellent. I couldn't want for better in-laws. I miss my nieces and nephews and my friends and the stuff that they do, but we talk on the phone a lot. My mom and my brother have been here a few times."

❀

Helen (nee Wheatley) Penney was born in Derbyshire, England, and graduated as a SRN in 1990 from Nottingham School of Nursing, England. She completed midwifery as a SCM from Queen's Medical Centre, Nottingham, in 1992 and immigrated to work as a midwife at the hospital in St. Anthony in 1997.

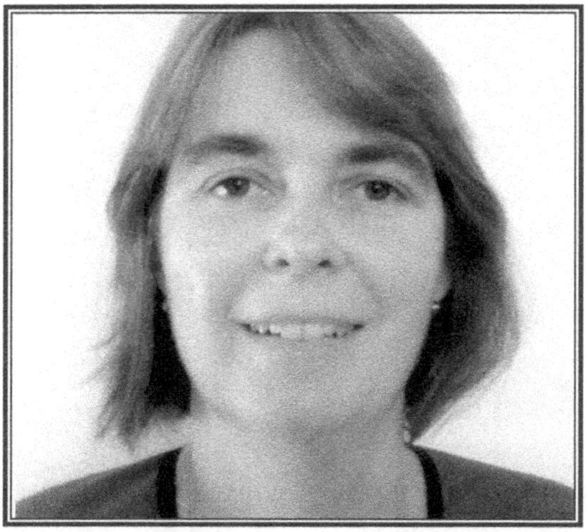

VEREENA (AEGERTER) EBSARY

1999

"In the end, one of the reasons we came back was that not all societies are like this society. I find the people here are very open and very helpful. It is awful to say this, but I don't think my own people are as welcoming to foreigners as people here are."

"When I finished training, my friend and I took time off and drove across Canada. We ended up in Newfoundland, where I met my husband, who was a tour guide at Cape Spear. I returned home but we kept in touch for four years. Then my husband moved to Switzerland for three years until we came here in 1999. We always planned to come to Newfoundland but I knew I wouldn't qualify for a work visa as a regular nurse. Doing midwifery was my way to get a work visa because then I could work as a midwife in St. Anthony or Goose Bay. Also we planned to buy one of the redundant lighthouses here, and Cape Bauld lighthouse, off Quirpon on the Northern Peninsula, became available in '98. We bid on it but didn't get it. Then I got a job in obstetrics at St. Anthony hospital and we moved here, although my husband is from St. John's.

"When we lived in Switzerland, we travelled to Newfoundland every summer and I had a chance to speak to somebody from Human Resources in the hospital in St. Anthony. On my first visit the HR manager was very discouraging and said I was better off staying where I was because at the time nobody was getting a job here. Then one summer I met the head midwife and found out there was a job opening here.

"I went through a lot to get here because I was afraid to come with just my regular schooling. I took a test from a place in Philadelphia which offered an out-of-country nursing test to see if you knew enough nursing to work in North America. I passed the exam, which gave me courage to think I could probably work in nursing here. I also had to do a proficiency test in English, but language wasn't a problem because living with my husband and my visits to Newfoundland made the difference language-wise. My nursing program in Switzerland included everything, which was why I was eligible to do nursing here. I had to write the RN exams but I could work on a temporary licence for six months before writing them, which was good because it gave me time to get used to nursing here. I had to know all topics but I had been a general nurse for seven years and understood the content, only the language was different.

"When I first came I was enchanted with the place and took a trip up the Labrador Coast on the *Northern Ranger*. I travelled with somebody who did research on the coast for Grenfell, so she took me into all the nursing stations. I met the nurses and thought it was a wonderful place to work. I have only worked in St. Anthony hospital and it's different from working in Switzerland in so many ways, but hard to define. It's funny how things that are healthy in one place might be unhealthy in another. You think the way you've been educated is how it should be, then you go somewhere else and things are done differently. When I came here I was amazed about handwashing. In Switzerland every nurse carried a bottle of hand disinfectant in her uniform pocket and we always had to spray. Everybody's hands were raw from alcohol use. It was crazy! Then I came here and that didn't exist. We only did handwashing, and I couldn't believe it! We didn't have any more infections here than where I worked in Switzerland. We had lots of mastitis there, but I haven't seen a mastitis case here yet. It's amazing!

"Taped reports were also different because we always did shift handovers person-to-person. I found it really hard to learn the medications here. It was a big challenge! Also, when I came St. Anthony still had the old crank beds, which really surprised me. And I couldn't get over giving bedtime snacks to patients! My husband told me about growing up and having mug-ups before going to bed, but that was the first I ever heard of it. Also everybody here drank ice water in such a cold climate, where back home they drink warm herbal teas. The language differences were hard at first and sometimes I still find it hard to understand the people from Labrador. But a nurse from St. John's who worked here told me she had a hearing test because she thought she couldn't understand because she didn't hear well. That made me feel better!

"Here I work as a midwife and an RN, but it's mostly RN work. In the past four or five years we've had between 110 and 130 deliveries, which are not many per midwife. We might each average 15 deliveries in a good year. Midwifery work here is very nice because we work independently, although we have obstetricians and there aren't many places where you can do that. In Switzerland you can work independently as a midwife, but you don't have doctors to back you up, or you can work in a hospital setting but are not as independent. It's wonderful here because it's like a birthing centre with an obstetrician in the background. It is special and a really great service for the women.

"I have been back to Switzerland and we have discussed going back. When our first daughter was two, we moved to Switzerland. I had a job and my husband's job was to look after our child. Luckily I took a year's leave of absence from St. Anthony and didn't quit because we found it really difficult when we went back. We were in the heart of Europe and could travel, which is one thing we don't have here. But there were crowds of people and the things that go with that. Before we went to Switzerland I became a Canadian, which made it possible for me to come back. Another reason we came back was that not all societies are like this one. The people here are very open and helpful. It's awful to say, but I don't think my own people are as welcoming to foreigners as the people here. My parents have been here several times. Last summer was the first where we didn't have people visiting. We always have visitors and they are amazed by the beauty of this place— so much space and it's really lovely. We came back, which is nice, and I think this is it."

＊

Verena (nee Aegerter) Ebsary was born in Brugg, Switzerland. She graduated in 1992 from Schweiz Pflegerinnen-schule, Zurich, Switzerland. She completed midwifery as a SCM in Switzerland in 1999 in preparation for immigration to St. Anthony.

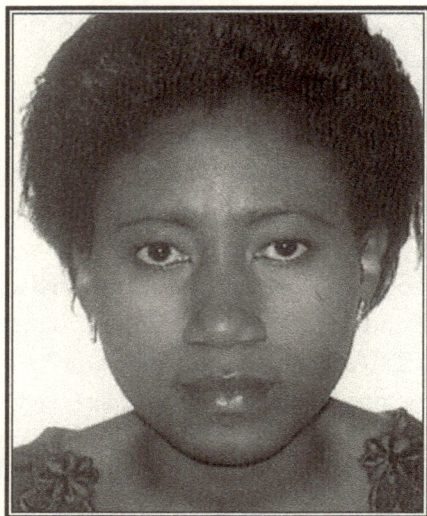

LOLA (ADEGBULU) ADEAGBO

❋

2007

"I saw an advert that Grenfell Health was coming to England to interview nurses. I asked, 'Where is Canada?' I heard about Canada, that it was a nice place with no crime … I needed to change my environment because of my children."

"I worked in England for about three years and came here in 2007. Finding out about Newfoundland came from God because it wasn't planned. My friends wanted me to come to America and I had started the process to do the exam when I saw an advert in *Nursing Times* that Grenfell Health was coming to England to interview nurses. I asked myself, 'Where is Canada?' I heard about Canada, that it was a nice place with no crime. In England, especially London, the crime rate is very high, and I needed to change my environment because London is not a good place to raise children.

"I was supposed to be on duty the day of the interview and didn't think I could make it. I looked for someone to cover my shift but couldn't find anyone, so I thought I'd let the interview go. I was called in to cover a night shift but told them I couldn't because I was on duty the next morning, which was the interview day. But a colleague said, 'You do the night shift and I'll cover your early shift.' I did that and went to the interview from there. The IGA staff had my credentials and when they saw my CV, they said, 'Oh, you're a midwife.' I never worked as a midwife in England because of the litigation problems there and I didn't want any problems. The staff asked, 'Why don't you come as a midwife,' but I said, 'No, I don't want to practice midwifery. I prefer being a nurse.' They said okay and gave me the website for ARNNL to get registered. ARNNL told me the requirements and that I had to do the IELTS (International English Language Testing System) English exam. I did it and passed. I sent home for my transcripts and documents and my mom did that for me. It took about eight months to get registered and get everything done. I sent my application to the high commission in England, and when the result came back, my husband and I came to Newfoundland. I was 22 weeks pregnant when I came and my baby was born here in July.

"Nursing is almost the same as it was in Nigeria and England, but some things are different. Here, some nurses call the doctor, who prescribes on the phone, and they give the treatment and write things for the doctor. Nurses don't do that in England. Even if the doctor tells you something on the phone you don't do it until the doctor documents it. In Nigeria nursing is really different. There, if you try to give a patient a medication and she says she isn't ready to take it, you tell her that if she doesn't take the medication, it's better if she went home and nursed herself. But in England it was a different experience. There you passed the medication to the patient and if she refused, you wrote refused and discarded the medication.

"I work in OBS here, which is a combination of OBS and pediatrics. We have a nice apartment very near work. At times I don't know what the weather is like because I don't have to go outside. I step out into a corridor that goes straight into the hospital and down to my ward.

"The people here have made us feel at home and are so friendly. Even on my ward, they are friendly. I understand people when I'm looking at their mouths, but if I'm not looking at them I can't really understand because of the accent and they talk very fast. I think they have the same problem with my accent because when I speak, they say, 'Sorry, pardon.' But I'm getting used to them. I'm so happy with the community here in St. Anthony. I'm very familiar with the environment and I attend the Pentecostal church.

"When we got here this guy picked us up on a bus. We were the only black people, so as soon as he saw us, he knew we were the ones and came over. When people in the community see us they ask, 'Are you a doctor?' because any black person who comes to St. Anthony is a doctor. For us it is unusual to be different and not from the same ethnic background as the community because London is jam-packed with black people and London accepts anybody."

✳

Funmilola (Lola) (nee Adegbulu) Adeagbo was born in Nigeria and graduated from Ondo State School of Nursing, Akure, Nigeria, in 1999 as a SRN. She completed midwifery in Nigeria in 2001 and immigrated to London before coming to the hospital in St. Anthony in 2007.

Conclusion

OVERSEAS RECRUITMENT OF NURSES provided much-needed human resources within the provincial health care system. Our research project was intended to document this piece of the history of nursing in Newfoundland and Labrador, but it has achieved much more. The experiences the nurses described not only shed light on the challenges they encountered in the workplace, but the challenges they faced with the lifestyle and culture of the province. The stories also revealed the realities of life in Newfoundland and Labrador, such as the difficult socio-economic circumstances in some regions of the province. They reflected life in the province as much as they did the experiences of nursing in the community.

Nurses coming to Newfoundland and Labrador saw it as a short-term venture. They came on work permits and contracted to work for a specific time period with the intent of returning home at the end of their contract. Making a permanent move to the province or to Canada was not a motivator for the majority except for those who immigrated with their spouses. These nurses came for both adventure and the opportunity to travel. As you read the stories, it is clear that this spirit motivated these nurses. Most had no knowledge of where Newfoundland and Labrador was, what it was about, or what was expected of them. Travelling to the province was the easy piece; once they got to Newfoundland and Labrador, the adventure started when they boarded yellow buses, canoes, or beaver planes to get to their final destination.

Their biggest challenge in nursing practice was the different names for drugs and equipment and the different perception of what was and what was not nursing. Their acceptance depended on where and when they went. For example, the nurses who went to St. Anthony assimilated into a group that was very much like themselves, whereas nurses who came to St. John's encountered differing reactions. In some cases the nurses were very supportive and in other cases they encountered harsh realities. In rural areas they were embraced by the community, whereas in urban areas they were often left to fend for themselves. In rural communities people readily welcomed the nurse and involved them in the life of the community. But in urban areas they generally socialized within their own group.

This group of nurses clearly adapted to the lifestyle and culture and spoke very highly about the kindness of the people. Some adapted quicker than others. Their struggles with the dialects, language, customs, food and the weather were individual and often depended on where they arrived. Towards the end of the interviews, many did acknowledge that they had adopted many of the characteristics of Newfoundlanders that caused them frustration in the beginning.

While many view Newfoundland and Labrador as their home and feel they have strong ties to the place, it is also very important that they maintain strong ties with family and former colleagues, particularly those from the UK.

Those who stayed became enmeshed in the community they came to nurse. They were really committed to the health of the people in the community where they lived. In addition to encountering some very difficult nursing situations they weren't prepared for, they also had to deal with very challenging environmental, communication and transportation issues. Yet they took to the lifestyle. This is what separated nurses who stayed from those who returned to their native country or moved on to further travel. Newfoundland and Labrador have benefited as much as the nursing community because these nurses opted to make a life and career in the province. They made (and are making) a tremendous contribution to nursing and health care because they stayed. Their accounts reflect the strong attachment they have for their adopted home.

Once again, worldwide nursing shortages are being felt in health care, and nursing recruitment in foreign countries has become a strategy to deal with them. These stories provide some insight into issues and challenges encountered by nurses who immigrated, as well as those faced by the broader health care community. Health care professionals and institutions weren't always prepared to give immigrating nurses what they needed when they arrived. By telling their stories, these nurses may have helped the nursing community, professional licensing bodies, and local employers prepare for and work with employees who were trained differently and who bring with them a new way of thinking. In telling their stories, they will have helped future nurses adapt to the reality of living and working away from home. ❧

Acknowledgements

This research was supported by a grant from the Associated Medical Services Inc. (AMS). AMS was established in 1936 by Dr. Jason Hannah as a pioneer prepaid not-for-profit health care organization in Ontario. With the advent of Medicare, AMS became a charitable organization supporting innovations in academic medicine and health services, specifically the history of medicine and health care, as well as innovations in health professional education and bioethics.

The authors wish to thank Memorial University School of Nursing (MUNSON) for the Research Award which facilitated completion of the interviews province wide. We also thank Joanne Smith-Young, Nursing Research Unit Coordinator at MUNSON, for transcribing the interviews and participating in the data analysis; Renee Lawrence for collecting documents from participants; and a special thank you to all the nurses throughout the province who agreed to be interviewed.

www.ingramcontent.com/pod-product-compliance
Lightning Source LLC
Chambersburg PA
CBHW022005080426
42733CB00007B/479